MIDWIFERY PRACTICE:

Core Topics 2

Edited by

Jo Alexander, Valerie Levy
and *Carolyn Roth*

First published 1997 by
MACMILLAN PRESS LTD
Houndmills, Basingstoke, Hampshire RG21 6XS
and London
Companies and representatives
throughout the world

ISBN 0-333-69627-1 paperback

A catalogue record for this book is available
from the British Library.

This book is printed on paper suitable for recycling and
made from fully managed and sustained forest sources.

10 9 8 7 6 5 4 3 2
07 06 05 04 03 02 01 00 99

Editing and origination by
Aardvark Editorial, Mendham, Suffolk

Printed and bound in Great Britain by
Antony Rowe Ltd
Chippenham, Wiltshire

*This volume is dedicated with thanks and
affection to Sarah Roch, to wish her well in her
(extremely active) retirement*

Contents

Other volumes in the Midwifery Practice series

■ **Midwifery practice: Core topics 1**   ISBN 0-333-66320-9

Rosemary Currell: The organisation of maternity care
Greta Curtis: Preconception care
Jennifer Wilson: Antenatal risk assessment
Colin Rees: Antenatal education, health promotion and the midwife
Elsa Montgomery: Fetal wellbeing: the intrauterine environment and ensuing legal and clinical issues
Jane Denton: Pregnancy after treatment for infertility
Helen R. Minns: Women with learning disabilities: the midwife's role
Tansy M. Cheston: Pre-eclampsia
Kathleen King: Marketing midwifery services

■ **Midwifery practice: a research-based approach**   ISBN 0-333-57617-9

Mavis Kirkham: Communication in midwifery
Elsa Montgomery: Iron and vitamin supplementation during pregnancy
Gillian Halksworth: Exercise and pregnancy
Joanne Whelton: Fetal medicine
Louise Silverton: The elderly primigravida
Paul Summersgill: Couvade – the retaliation of marginalised fathers
Mary Kensington: Safer motherhood – a midwifery challenge
Valerie Fletcher: Pain and the neonate
Jean A. Ball: Workload measurement in midwifery
Robert Dingwall: Negligence litigation research and the practice of midwifery

■ **Aspects of midwifery practice**   ISBN 0-333-61956-0

Sally Spedding, Joan Wilson, Sarah Wright and Alan Jackson: Nutrition for pregnancy and lactation
Rosaline Steele: Midwifery care in the first stage of labour
Elaine Carty: Disability, pregnancy and parenting
Terri Coates: Shoulder dystocia
Catherine Siney: Drug addicted mothers
Carolyn Roth: HIV and pregnancy
Jennifer Sleep: Postnatal perineal care revisited
Susan L. Smith: Neonatal hypoglycaemia
Sally Marchant and Jo Garcia: Routine clinical care in the immediate postnatal period

Contributors to this volume

Carol Bates MA, RN, RM, ADM, PGCEA
Professional Development Programme Coordinator, Education & Practice
Development, Royal College of Midwives
Carol Bates was Director of Midwifery Education at the Obstetric Hospital, University College Hospitals, London from 1992 until 1996. The topic of her MA dissertation was a feminist perspective of motherhood.

Chris Bewley MSc, BEd, RGN, RM, ADM
Set Leader for Midwifery Education at Middlesex Hospital
Chris Bewley has written previously about domestic violence and pregnancy, medical complications and midwifery, and midwifery education issues.

Rona Campbell BSc, MSc, PhD
Lecturer, Health Services Research, Department of Social Medicine,
University of Bristol
Rona Campbell has had a long-standing interest in the evaluation of maternity services in general and the evidence on place of birth in particular, and has written widely on these matters. With social scientist Jo Garcia she has recently written a book on how to evaluate the organisation of midwifery care.

Tansy M Cheston RGN, RM
Midwifery Sister, Day Assessment Unit, The John Radcliffe Hospital, Oxford
Tansy Cheston is currently a practising midwifery sister particularly concerned with high-risk pregnancies in Oxford. Many of the women in her care have diabetes. Tansy has also written on pre-eclampsia for a previous volume in this series.

Rona McCandlish RM, RMN, RGN, BA
Research Midwife, The National Perinatal Epidemiology Unit, Oxford
Rona McCandlish is at present co-ordinating a large randomised controlled trial about perineal care during the second stage of labour. Her other research interests include management of perineal trauma, and the use of immersion in water during labour and birth.

Sue McDonald RN, RM, CHN, BApp.Sc
Midwifery and Nursing Researcher, King Edward Memorial Hospital,
Centre for Women's Health, Western Australia
Having recently completed a PhD on the active management of labour, Sue McDonald co-reviews this topic for the Cochrane Library. She is currently

involved in a randomised controlled trial, comparing epidural versus continuous midwifery support for pain relief in labour.

Cliff Roberts MSc, BSc (Hons), PGDE, RGN
Lecturer in Clinical Neurophysiology and Midwifery Studies, RCN Institute, London
Specialist interest in the clinical neurophysiology/pharmacology of pain applied to the care of children, adults, critical care and midwifery.

Jane Rogers BA, SRN, RM, DPSM
Midwife in clinical practice and Research Midwife, Hinchingbrooke Hospital, Huntingdon
With Juliet Wood, Jane Rogers instigated and conducted the Hinchingbrooke Third Stage Trial.

Maxine Wallis-Redworth RN, RM, ADM, PGCEA, BSc (Hons)
Midwifery Tutor and Co-ordinator of the Clinical Academic Unit – Neonates, European Institute of Health and Medical Sciences, University of Surrey
Maxine Wallis-Redworth is currently registered for a PhD within the European Institute of Health and Medical Sciences.

Juliet Wood BSc (Hons), RGN, RM, ADM
Midwifery Sister (Research and Clinical Practice), Hinchingbrooke Hospital, Huntingdon, Cambridgeshire
Juliet Wood works in clinical practice and, with her colleague Jane Rogers, instigated and co-ordinated the Hinchingbrooke Third Stage Trial.

Carole Yearley RN, RM, ADM, PCEA, MSc (Medical Anthropology)
Senior Lecturer in Midwifery
Carole Yearley is a midwife teacher and is currently the Scheme Leader for the Family Planning course in Hertfordshire. She has a particular interest in fertility and women's sexual health and is also interested in the impact of culture on health, sickness and other life events.

Foreword

Having been in at the conception, birth and early development of this series, I was particularly delighted to be asked to write this foreword to Core Topics 2, the first volume to be published since I retired and relinquished my joint editorship.

The series is now in its formative years, and this new volume demonstrates its continued commitment to fulfil the major original aim of the series, which was to provide busy practising midwives with well-evaluated, relevant research firmly linked to real-life clinical practice.

This new book is both exciting and stimulating. It has splendid breadth as well as considerable depth of professional knowledge. It traverses the whole spectrum from the fascinating feminist viewpoint to the traditionally (and mostly male!), obstetric-centred world of birth emergencies and the medicalisation of normal labour.

The anthropological perspective is particularly welcome as it provides a gateway to far broader scientific learning relating to culture and rituals in the amazing adaptation process women experience through pregnancy to parenthood. The vital insights obtained through this discipline can be sensibly linked to the real practicalities of providing sensitive, loving maternity care for the whole family.

The main thrust of the text is focused on labour, and I was enthralled to find such a healthy balance between the 'scientific' element of the research content, and the 'art' of midwifery in the distilled clinical wisdom. A splendid amalgam! As Shakespeare said in *The Taming of the Shrew*, 'O, this learning! What a thing it is!'.

Despite some contentious topics, I feel proud that my profession now looks much more objectively at these areas of practice that tend to cause interprofessional dissent. This book gives a well-balanced and largely unbiased evaluation of current research, and hopefully this approach will become the norm for all professions involved in childbirth.

We must keep reminding ourselves that some of today's 'pearls' of research wisdom are tomorrow's errors, and be ever vigilant in keeping abreast of new data to underpin safe clinical practice fit for the next millennium!

I look forward to more volumes in this series for, as the Greek philosopher Solon said, 'I grow old ever learning'.

Sarah Roch

Preface

Core Topics 1, the sixth volume in the *Midwifery Practice* series, marked a watershed in our endeavours to provide practical, readable research-based texts for busy practitioners at an affordable price. We have listened to our 'consumers' and continue to strive to meet their varying needs in a rapidly changing care environment. Chapters retain the proven structure described below. The contributors address topical concerns as well as reviewing and updating some of the fundamental subject areas so important to midwifery. Again, we have sought a balance between core topics and contemporary issues in this volume, and we would welcome suggestions for future volumes.

Since beginning this series, it has become generally easier for midwives to access databases such as the Cochrane Collaborative Pregnancy and Childbirth Database and the MIRIAD Midwifery Research Database. However, practitioners do still benefit from having access to sound, well-referenced texts that address their needs and review a spread of relevant and up to date reference material. For some, this satisfies their needs, while for others it provides a springboard to the achievement of higher-level knowledge and research activity. As editors, we are committed to remaining firmly rooted in clinical practice, appealing both to those with limited time and to those wishing to investigate topics further.

Our contributors have delighted us with their meticulous work and willingness to meet our aspirations. Their critical appraisals of the literature will stimulate the reader seeking to evaluate different research approaches, and all midwives should find much to enhance their evidence-based practice. Women using the maternity services are increasingly knowledgeable and expect midwives to be properly equipped, both practically and academically. Getting the balance right is not easy, but we hope that this series will continue to make a useful contribution in this arena, encouraging education and practice to stay welded together and jointly driving clinical research.

Finally, we would like to thank our publishers, especially our outstanding publishers' editor Richenda Milton-Thompson, and Carrie Walker who has recently joined us as copy editor.

The above is largely unchanged since its appearance in *Core Topics 1* since when Sarah Roch has retired from her editing role and Carolyn Roth has most ably taken her place. We are grateful to Sarah for her enormous input into the series so far.

Jo Alexander
Valerie Levy
Carolyn Roth

■ Common structure of the chapters

In fulfilment of the aims of the series, each chapter follows a common structure:

1. The introduction offers a digest of the contents;

2. 'It is assumed that you are already aware of the following... ' establishes the prerequisite knowledge and experience assumed of the reader;

3. The main body of the chapter then reviews and analyses the most appropriate and important research literature currently available;

4. The 'Recommendations for clinical practice' offer suggestions for sound clinical practice, based on the author's interpretation of the literature;

5. The 'Practice check' enables professionals to examine their own practice and the principles and policies influencing their work;

6. Bibliographic sources are covered under 'References' and 'Suggested further reading'.

■ Suggested further reading on research

Cormack DFS (ed.) 1996 The research process in nursing, 3rd edn. Blackwell Science, Oxford
Couchman W, Dawson J 1995 Nursing and healthcare research, 2nd edn. Scutari Press, London
Distance Learning Centre modules 1987–95 Research awareness: a programme for nurses, midwives and health visitors, Units 1–11. South Bank University, London
Hicks C 1990 Research and statistics: a practical introduction for nurses. Prentice Hall, Hemel Hempstead
Parahoo, K 1997 Nursing research: principles, process, issues. Macmillan, Basingstoke
Polit DF, Hungler BP 1995 Nursing research: principles and methods, 5th edn. JB Lippincott, Philadelphia

Chapter 1

Place of birth reconsidered

Rona Campbell

The maternity services aim to help women achieve a favourable outcome to a normal physiological process. Because the main concern is not illness but an important and life-changing event, the services cannot be solely concerned with physical health but must also respond to the social, emotional, educational and economic needs of the mother. ...One fixed pattern of care will not be suitable for everyone and the provision of a service which is flexible, adaptable and readily available is a pre-requisite to success.

(Royal College of Midwives 1987)

Women should be encouraged to have babies in the larger and properly consultant staffed units of district general hospitals, which can offer the whole range of obstetric, paediatric and supporting services necessary to cope with any emergencies at the time when the life of an infant is most frail and when the life of the mother may be threatened.

(House of Commons 1985)

Both of these statements, made in the mid 1980s, reflect two very different perspectives on childbirth. The former sees childbirth as a 'normal physiological process' which requires that a variety of maternity care options be available if all women's needs are to be taken into account. The latter characterises birth as hazardous to mother and child and only to be conducted in a hospital setting that has the 'supporting services necessary to cope with any emergencies'. For much of the past 45 years, it is the medicalised view of childbirth which has guided policy on place of birth, although the question of where women should give birth and whether certain locations are safer than others has been argued over for centuries in the UK (Donnison 1977; Smith 1979). Until recently opinion, rather than evidence, and the genuine difficulties in interpreting the sometimes meagre and unrefined evidence available have proved significant obstacles to resolving this debate and arriving at rational policies.

This chapter begins by charting the official sanctioning and encouragement of a move from home to hospital birth and the recent reversal of this

1

policy. A review of the research evidence on the relative safety of birth at home compared with that in an institutional setting, which follows, calls into question the extent to which past policy, pursued on grounds of safety, was justified. Research evidence relating to alternatives to delivery in a consultant-led unit are discussed together with issues of choice, cost and selection for delivery outside hospital.

■ It is assumed that you are already aware of the following:

- The different places in which women can give birth;
- The definitions of 'perinatal mortality rate' and 'maternal mortality rate';
- The difference between observational and experimental research.

■ Policy on place of birth

There have been several distinct phases in policy making on the place of birth. The first, which existed from before the turn of the century and lasted until the mid 1940s, was characterised by a consensus that the majority of women could give birth safely at home and that hospital delivery was required only for women with complications. During this phase, there was also a recognition that women without complications might require institutional delivery, not for clinical reasons, but in order that they might give birth and recuperate afterwards in a more congenial setting than most people's homes afforded at the time. This idea particularly took root in the period after World War I because of the poor and overcrowded housing conditions prevailing in urban areas. Concerns about high rates of maternal mortality did not result in pressure for greater institutional delivery but did lead to the formation of a national maternity service (Peretz 1990). This was based in local authority public health departments, which were led by a medical officer of health. The backbone of this service was the domiciliary midwife, with GP and specialist obstetric care available if required.

World War II and the introduction of the NHS resulted in a number of changes that increased the number of births in hospital. The physical damage and social disruption of World War II resulted in many more births taking place in institutional settings. There was also a change in attitude towards domiciliary delivery. The introduction of the NHS concentrated power in the hands of the hospital consultant, and, for the next 45 years, consultant obstetricians enjoyed considerable influence over policy on the place of birth.

A definite shift in policy making began in the mid 1940s, when the Royal College of Obstetricians and Gynaecologists (RCOG) (1944) proposed that

70 per cent of births should take place in hospital. This was adopted as official policy in 1959 (Ministry of Health 1959). In a relatively short time, medical opinion had changed from a position that only a minority of births required hospital delivery to the stance that the majority of births should take place there. From the mid 1950s, as Figure 1.1 illustrates, there was a sharp rise in the number of births taking place in hospital, so that the target of 70 per cent hospital delivery was achieved by 1964.

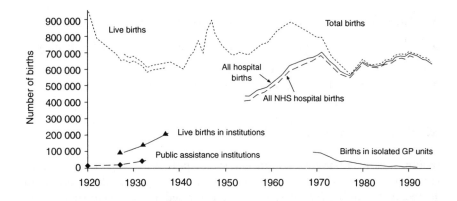

Note: Isolated GP units were not identified separately after 1992

Source: Office for National Statistics, Birth statistics, Series FM 1

Figure 1.1 Births in institutions, England and Wales, 1920–95

From the mid 1960s, the total number of births began falling. This coincided with a reduction in the length of stay in hospital after birth. An oversupply of hospital maternity beds thus became a real possibility. This problem was averted when a government committee took up another proposal, which had been made earlier by the RCOG (1954), and recommended 'that sufficient facilities should be provided to allow for 100 per cent hospital delivery'. The committee went on to justify this by stating that 'The greater safety of hospital confinement for mother and child justifies this objective' (Standing Maternity and Midwifery Advisory Committee 1970). This policy stance was sustained by successive government committees and ministers until the beginning of the 1990s, but, despite this, '100 per cent hospital delivery' was never quite attained and the proportion of births taking place at home remained at about 1 per cent of all births throughout most of the 1980s, with a slight but steady increase at the end of the decade.

Other developments were taking place during the 1980s which substantially increased the pressure for change. Groups seeking to represent the interests of consumers campaigned vigorously for a more pluralistic pattern of maternity care. The positions of various professional groups involved also became more clearly differentiated, with the Royal College of Midwives and the Royal College of General Practitioners supporting the case for planned delivery outside hospital obstetric units (President of the Royal College of Obstetricians and Gynaecologists *et al* 1992). In response to these developments, the House of Commons Health Committee conducted an inquiry into the maternity services and came to some rather different conclusions from those of previous committees when it concluded that 'the policy of encouraging all women to give birth in hospital cannot be justified on grounds of safety' (House of Commons Health Committee 1992). Still this view was not accepted by the government, and another committee, the Expert Maternity Group, under the chairmanship of Baroness Cumberlege, Parliamentary Under Secretary of State for Health, was set up to look into the matter further. In its report, *Changing childbirth,* the Expert Maternity Group also concluded that 'There is no clear statistical evidence that having their babies away from general hospital maternity units is less safe for women with uncomplicated pregnancies'. It recommended that 'Women should receive clear, unbiased advice and be able to choose where they would like their baby to be born' (DoH 1993). This report was initially issued as a consultation document but was subsequently accepted by the government and became official policy. The direct involvement of a government minister in *Changing childbirth* guaranteed the report a high profile and has ensured that considerable efforts are being made to see that its recommendations are implemented (Jackson 1996).

■ The research evidence

The research evidence, which was cited as justification for this radical change in policy, is complex. When the initial booking is made for a place of birth, not only is the delivery location selected, but decisions are often also being made about the pattern of antenatal and postnatal care and about the lead professional, that is, the midwife, GP or obstetrician. The nature of the care available also varies according to the place of birth. Women booking for delivery at home are more likely to achieve continuity of care than are those giving birth in hospital. Likewise, the social relationships between the childbearing woman and her carers are different when the birth occurs in the woman's home, where she is in control and her carers are guests. The issue of control is important because it is linked to better emotional outcomes (Green *et al* 1988). As the sort of care available at different locations, and the type of staff providing it, varies considerably from country to country in ways which might affect outcomes, only studies undertaken in the UK will be considered in this chapter.

The mortalities of mothers and babies have been the main outcome measures used as indicators of the relative safety of different places of birth.

The use of such apparently straightforward indices is not, however, without its problems. For the latter half of the 20th century, maternal deaths have been so rare as to make statistical comparisons impossible. Rates of stillbirth and neonatal death have also declined substantially and are now sufficiently low in women with uncomplicated pregnancies as to make comparison difficult. Nevertheless, much of the evidence on safety and place of birth comes from studies of perinatal mortality and is therefore included in the review of evidence that follows. Unfortunately, simply comparing rates of perinatal deaths in one location with those in another, as many studies have done, can be misleading if factors such as the proportions of babies with lethal congenital abnormalities, the proportion of babies weighing less than 2500 g and whether the death occurred before or after the onset of labour are not taken into account.

Many of the studies comparing mortality by place of birth date from a time when mortality was much higher. Numbers of deaths are now so low that the focus has shifted to comparisons of morbidity, costs and parents' views. There is also a need to consider the question of equity, that is, are the maternity services that women want and need available to them?

■ Comparing birth in an institutional setting with birth at home

There has been a widespread belief that the decline in perinatal mortality resulted, at least in part, from the move towards hospital delivery (Maternity Services Advisory Committee 1984; House of Commons 1987). As the previous section has illustrated, policy was also predicated on the assumption that hospital was the safest place in which to give birth.

Findings from a number of detailed studies published in the late 1970s suggested that any association between perinatal mortality and a change in place of birth was coincidental rather than causal (Chalmers *et al* 1976; Barron *et al* 1977; Ashford 1978; Tew 1978). Furthermore, the proportion of births at home has increased from less than 1 per cent in 1987 to almost 2 per cent in 1994, but there has been no commensurate increase in perinatal mortality. Indeed, as Figure 1.2 illustrates, the perinatal mortality for all births at home has continued to decline.

Since 1975 the Office of Population Censuses and Surveys (OPCS), which has recently combined with other government statistical organisations to form the Office of National Statistics (ONS), has linked the death registration of any infant dying within the first year of life to its birth registration. This has enabled perinatal mortality rates by place of birth to be calculated. When these were first published in the late 1970s, considerable concern was expressed about the rise in perinatal mortality for births occurring at home. Indeed, a government committee was prompted to recommend the continued phasing-out of home delivery (Social Services Committee 1980).

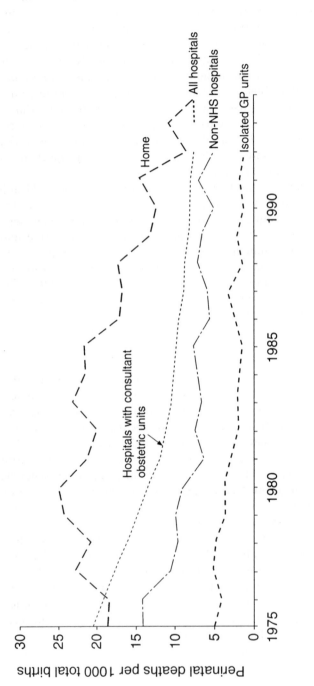

Source: Office for National Statistics.

Notes: 1. From 1993 onwards, no distinction was made between different types of hospital.
2. Stillbirths at 24–27 weeks of gestation have been excluded from perinatal mortality rates for October 1992 onwards.

Figure 1.2 Perinatal mortality by place of birth, England and Wales, 1975–94

It was misleading to draw this conclusion without qualification. Women giving birth at home may do so unintentionally. A national study of all home births in 1979 showed perinatal mortality for planned home births to be very low, at 4.1 per 1000 births. For parous women, the rate was even lower – 2.5 per 1000 (Campbell *et al* 1984). Rates for birth booked for delivery in consultant units but occurring at home were much higher, at 67.5 per 1000. Thus, an increase in the proportion of unplanned births at home relative to those planned to occur there was, almost certainly, the reason for the increase in overall perinatal mortality for birth at home (Tew 1981; Campbell *et al* 1984). The subsequent decline in this rate in the latter half of the 1980s suggests that the proportion of unplanned births at home has fallen.

A survey of perinatal mortality in the former Northern Regional Health Authority in England from 1981 until 1994 estimated a perinatal mortality rate of 1.7 per 1000 for planned home births. When deaths to women who had planned to give birth at home but who subsequently transferred into hospital in labour were included, the estimated rate was 4.8 per 1000, which was less than half the rate for the region as a whole (Northern Regional Perinatal Mortality Survey Coordinating Group 1996). The perinatal mortality rate for women who were booked for hospital delivery but gave birth at home was estimated to be between 45 and 54.3 per 1000. This suggests the persistence of patterns of perinatal mortality observed for home births occurring in 1979.

There have been no randomised trials comparing outcomes for home and hospital deliveries. In the past, it would have been theoretically possible to conduct such trials in order to determine whether there were differences in perinatal mortality. Because levels of mortality are now so low, particularly among those women who have uncomplicated pregnancies, the number required to participate in order to detect statistically significant differences in mortality is so great as to make such a trial impossible (Lilford 1987). While randomised comparisons could still examine other outcome measures, such as levels of breastfeeding and rates of postnatal depression, there is doubt over whether sufficient women would be willing to participate in such a trial (Dowswell *et al* 1996).

Most evidence comes from observational studies. Women at different risk of perinatal problems tend to give birth in different places, which makes it difficult to assess the extent to which differences in outcome are attributable to differences in the place of birth or to pre-existing differences. Therefore, some researchers have tried to take account of these selection biases when examining differences in mortality according to place of birth (Tew 1990; SJ Senn unpublished data).

Table 1.1 Births and perinatal mortality rates (PNMRs)
by labour prediction score (LPS) and place of birth, 1970

Level of risk	LPS	Number	%	Percentage of births		PNMR per 1000 births	
				Hospital	GP unit and home	Hospital	GP unit and home
Very low	0–1	7488	45.9	58.7	41.3	8.0	3.9*
Low	2	3723	22.8	68.8	31.2	17.9	5.2†
Moderate	3	2273	13.9	76.6	23.4	32.3	3.8‡
High	4–6	2417	14.7	84.0	16.0	53.2	15.5†
Very high	7–12	427	2.6	96.5	3.5	162.6	133.3

Significance of difference in rates: *p< 0.025; ‡p< 0.005; †p<0.001.

Source: Unpublished data from the British Births 1970 survey (Tew 1990).

The most important example of work of this kind was that undertaken by Marjorie Tew. She used mortality rates from a survey of births in Britain in 1970 and had them tabulated by a score that had been devised to reflect the predicted risk of complications in labour. As the data in Table 1.1 show, the level of perinatal mortality rose according to the level of predicted risk. When a comparison was made within risk categories between births taking place in hospital and births occurring at home or in GP maternity units, perinatal mortality was found to be significantly higher for hospital births at all but the highest level of risk (Tew 1990). Findings from this and other studies provide no evidence to support the commonly held view that, for all women, hospital is the safest place in which to give birth. It is not possible to conclude, however, that birth at home is safer because doubts remain about whether all selection biases can ever be controlled for.

■ Midwife-led care and place of birth

Midwives have always undertaken the majority of births whatever the location. Regrettably, because research and policy making have rarely involved midwives in any meaningful way, this fact has not always been acknowledged. Happily, this situation is changing. Julia Allison's reconstruction of the work of the district midwifery service in Nottingham from 1948 to 1972 is a good example of the trend towards midwives undertaking and publishing their own research (Allison 1996). During this period in Nottingham, a substantial proportion (42 per cent) of women had midwife-led care at home. As the data in Table 1.2 indicate, the mortality of babies born at home was substantially lower than that of those born in hospital. These results were achieved for women who often lived in materially impoverished circumstances.

The lower mortality rate for births occurring at home compared with hospital births has previously been attributed to the fact that only those women thought to be unlikely to experience complications were booked for delivery at home. Julia Allison's work casts considerable doubt on the adequacy of this explanation. Using the registers of 14 midwives who undertook almost one-fifth of all deliveries in the period 1955–72, she has been able to estimate that, on the grounds of maternal age, parity, multiple birth and gestational age, more than half of the women giving birth at home did not fulfil the criteria used from 1967 onwards in Nottingham. Moreover, births occurring at home to women who were booked for delivery in hospital, or those who were not booked anywhere for delivery, were included in the statistics as a home birth. The perinatal mortality rates for these groups were high, at 75 and 142 per 1000 births respectively. Correspondingly, the outcome of births to women booked for birth at home but transferred to hospital during labour would have been counted towards that of hospital births. Although Julia Allison was unable to calculate the mortality for this latter group, she has demonstrated that, contrary to what has generally been assumed, the number of women having unbooked births at home was greater than the number of women booked for delivery at home but transferred to hospital during labour.

Table 1.2 Live and stillbirths to Nottingham city residents by place of birth, 1955–72

Year	Live births		Stillbirths		Stillbirth rate	
	Home	Hospital	Home	Hospital	Home	Hospital
1955–57	8011	7770	87	269	10.9	34.6
1958–60	8672	8372	66	286	7.6	34.1
1961–63	9354	9172	59	285	6.1	31.0
1964–66	8062	10406	39	297	5.2	28.5
1967–69	5987	11409	32	242	5.3	21.1
1970–72	3682	11162	23	181	6.2	16.2
Total	43768	58291	306	1560	6.9	27.6

Source: City of Nottingham Medical Officer of Health Reports 1955–72 (Allison, 1996)

This work provides evidence that the care provided by the domiciliary midwifery service was, contrary to official claims at the time, far from unsafe. It also corroborates other work (Tew 1990) suggesting that the higher perinatal mortality rates associated with delivery in consultant obstetric units compared with other places before the mid 1970s was not simply because women at higher risk of complications gave birth there, as has often been assumed.

Another important development in the past 10 years has been the introduction of midwife-led units. These have developed in a variety of different settings. Most seem to be integrated with a consultant obstetric unit, that is, sharing some facilities but having separate delivery rooms (MacVicar *et al* 1993; Hundley *et al* 1994; Turnbull *et al* 1996). At least one midwife-led unit has been opened in a district general hospital without consultant units (Campbell & Macfarlane 1996), and one operates in a small community hospital (Ayres 1996). As their name suggests, they all share the same defining characteristic, which is that they are run by midwives. Medical assistance is sought only when the midwives deem it necessary. In some ways, these units are reminiscent of maternity homes built during the 1920s, which were staffed by midwives, medical help being called in only when required (Local Government Board 1918).

To date in the UK, there have been three randomised trials comparing outcomes for midwife-led units with those for conventional consultant obstetric care. No significant differences in mortality or life-threatening morbidity were found in any of the trials, but, because such outcomes are rare in women at low risk of obstetric complications, trials involving much larger numbers would be required before such differences could be detected (MacVicar *et al* 1993; Hundley *et al* 1994; Turnbull *et al* 1996). All found some intervention rates to be higher in consultant-led care. Two trials reported levels of satisfaction to be higher among those allocated to midwife-led care (MacVicar *et al* 1993; Turnbull *et al* 1996). Greater continuity of care and midwife autonomy, which resulted in greater midwife satisfaction with midwife-led care, was reported in one trial (Hundley *et al* 1994). This trial also indicated that the introduction of midwife-led care resulted in a considerable increase in the cost per woman delivered. Transfer rates from midwife- to consultant-led care were high in all three trials, one third to one half of women transferring before delivery. A non-randomised comparison of women booked for delivery in a midwife-led unit sited in a district general hospital but some miles from a consultant obstetric unit, and a similar group of women booked for care in the consultant unit, found some differences in the patterns of care they received but no differences in outcome (Campbell & Macfarlane 1996).

■ GP-led units

GP-led units, like midwifery-led units, have developed in a variety of settings (Campbell 1990). Isolated GP maternity units that are not on the same hospital site as a consultant obstetric unit used to be identified in official birth statistics as 'NHS Hospital A', but this has been abandoned because the ONS does not have sufficient information for classifying maternity units (Macfarlane *et al* 1995). Perinatal mortality rates for births taking place in these units, published for England and Wales from 1975 until 1991 by the OCPS, indicate that the rate has always been low. They do not, however, represent the full picture as they do not include perinatal deaths of babies born to women who were booked for this type of care but were transferred to a consultant unit before the baby was born.

Four observational studies indicate that the overall perinatal mortality rate is not affected by the proportion of deliveries that take place in GP units (Fryer & Ashford 1972; Taylor *et al* 1980; Black 1982; Mugford unpublished data). A fifth study claimed to demonstrate that it was not as safe to book for an isolated GP unit as a consultant unit (Sangala *et al* 1990) but questions have been raised about the adequacy of the statistical analysis (Campbell & Macfarlane 1990; Charney 1990), and data for later years do not support the original conclusion (Wiltshire Healthcare Trust unpublished data). A review of all the studies published internationally comparing GP or family doctor care with that provided by obstetricians found that, in all but one case, the outcome was the same for both types of care (Zander & Klein 1989).

A number of studies have suggested that, for low-risk women, rates of intervention (Lowe *et al* 1987) and maternal morbidity (Taylor *et al* 1980) for those cared for in GP-led units are lower than for those cared for in consultant obstetric units. There is also evidence that women prefer this form of care (Taylor 1986).

■ Selection for and transfer to consultant-led care

Women do not always give birth in the place originally chosen. As a result of complications arising during pregnancy, a women may be rebooked for delivery in a consultant unit, or she may be transferred to hospital in labour. Studies (many dating from a time when rates of mortality were higher than at present) have shown mortality to be higher among those who transfer compared with those who remain at home (Rutter 1964; Hobbs & Acheson 1966a, 1966b; Hudson 1968; Woodall 1968; Golding & Peters 1988; Clarke *et al* 1993). Although it has been argued that this raised mortality is the result of adverse effects of obstetric intervention in hospital (Tew 1986), a more likely explanation is that those who transfer are at greater risk compared with those remaining at home.

Booking for delivery in places other than a consultant obstetric unit and subsequent transfer of booking are usually governed by selection criteria. These are often based on criteria developed during the 1950s to ensure that those most in need were able to secure a hospital delivery (Campbell & Macfarlane 1994). The ability of such criteria now to identify those women who may experience problems during labour and delivery has been questioned (Reynolds *et al* 1988).

Evidence from a number of fairly recent studies of GP- and midwife-led care points to a number of trends as far as transfers are concerned. Rates of antenatal transfer varied from 20 per cent (Young 1987) to 38 per cent (Hundley *et al* 1994), of those in labour from 6 per cent (Young 1987) to 21 per cent (MacVicar *et al* 1993) and of those after birth from 1 per cent (Prentice & Walton 1989) to 3 per cent (MacVicar *et al* 1993). A recent survey of home births gave an antenatal transfer rate for obstetric reasons of 15 per cent (excluding women who miscarried) and a rate of 15 per cent for transfers in labour (Davies *et al* 1996).

In addition, primiparous women are three to four times more likely to be transferred during labour (Davies *et al* 1987; Garrett *et al* 1987; Young 1987; Reynolds *et al* 1988; Prentice & Walton 1989). Transfer, either antenatally or intrapartum, appears to be more likely if the unit is immediately adjacent to a consultant obstetric unit (Garrett *et al* 1987; Young 1987; MacVicar *et al* 1993; Hundley *et al* 1994). However, if women can be temporarily transferred to consultant care while a problem is investigated, and then referred back to the type of care originally booked if the problem resolves, close proximity to a consultant unit need not result in very high rates of permanent transfer (Turnbull *et al* 1996).

The most common reasons for transfer before the onset of labour are pregnancy-induced hypertension and postmaturity. The complications which most frequently lead to transfer in labour are fetal distress and a delay in labour. Although we know from earlier studies that mortality associated with transfer was higher than for those who gave birth in the place intended, the small number of deaths reported in these more recent studies do not allow any conclusions to be drawn, and regrettably such data are not available nationally (Macfarlane *et al* 1995). Although transfer is sometimes equated with failure, recent work suggests that women who transfer to consultant-led care with their carer do not regret their original booking decision (Creasey 1994).

■ Morbidity and place of birth

A number of descriptive studies have suggested that mothers (Alment *et al* 1967) and babies (Chamberlain *et al* 1978; Jarvis *et al* 1985) cared for in a hospital setting experience higher rates of non-life-threatening morbidity, such as episiotomy and tearing in women, and a higher proportion of low Apgar scores in babies. Although the findings of these studies are of interest, it is not possible to assess the extent to which differences in morbidity are directly attributable to differences in place of birth as no attempt was made to control for selection biases.

To reduce the effects of selection, three studies compared morbidity in similar groups of women thought to be at low risk of developing complications who gave birth in different places. Two studies compared women booked for delivery in a consultant unit with women booked to deliver under the care of their GP at home (Shearer 1985) and in an integrated GP unit (Klein *et al* 1980). Both studies found that a higher proportion of babies born to women booked for consultant care had low Apgar scores, but in one of the studies, this difference was confined to nulliparous women (Klein *et al* 1983). A third study, contrasting the morbidity of those booked for delivery in an isolated GP unit with those giving birth in a consultant unit, did not find a significant difference in the proportion of babies with Apgar scores of less than 6. Meconium staining and intubation were, however, more common among the babies born to mothers booked for birth in the consultant unit (Garrett *et al* 1987; Lowe *et al* 1987). Shearer (1985) also reported a significantly lower rate of episiotomy among women booked for birth at home, but this difference was not reported in another study (Garrett *et al* 1987; Lowe *et al* 1987).

The problems of selection bias when contrasting morbidity rates associated with different places of birth have been overcome in more recent evaluations of midwifery-led units that have been undertaken as randomised trials. (These are discussed in more detail in a subsequent section.) However, like the earlier studies discussed above, the number of women participating in these trials was such that they do not provide sufficient comparative data on the more serious but rare conditions from which to draw any conclusions.

■ Women's preferences

Probably because birth outside hospital has been discouraged for much of the past 30 years, there have, until recently, been few large-scale systematic investigations of women's preferences regarding place of birth (Campbell 1990). A survey manual designed to help service providers to assess women's views of maternity care, which was published by the OCPS in 1990, did not contain questions on whether a choice of place of birth was offered or on what options women would have liked in its standard questionnaires (Mason 1990). The issue was addressed only tangentially by including questions on whether women would have liked to have 'talked more about whether' they might have a home birth, domino delivery or choice of hospital.

All of the surveys of women who have experienced both home and hospital deliveries have found a strong preference for home birth (Gordon & Elias-Jones 1960; Alment *et al* 1967; Fleury 1967; Goldthorp & Richman 1974; O'Brien 1978). Most have involved opportunistic, non-random samples, and thus the findings may be unrepresentative. The same finding was, however, replicated in the one national survey to use random sampling (O'Brien 1978). There is, however, a further difficulty in interpreting these findings. Although all the studies were undertaken some time ago, the relatively small number of women who give birth at home may even then have contained a disproportionate number of women who opted for home birth, having been unhappy with a previous hospital birth.

During much of the last 15 years, fewer than 1 per cent of women giving birth had a home delivery. Asking women to make hypothetical choices about where they would like to give birth, in a situation in which home birth may be no longer thought of as an option, is problematic. Apart from those who have been dissatisfied with their care, most women tend to express a preference for whatever type of care they have had in the past (Jacoby &

Cartwright 1990). Thus it is not surprising that the vast majority of women now express a preference for hospital delivery (Johnson *et al* 1992). Nevertheless, there is evidence that considerably more women than those currently having a planned home birth would welcome this as a possible choice. As part of its work, the Expert Maternity Group commissioned MORI to undertake a survey of women who had recently given birth. Seventy-two per cent of respondents indicated that they would have liked the option of a system of care other than delivery in a consultant obstetric unit, 44 per cent said they would like the choice of a midwife-led domino delivery and 22 per cent favoured a home birth (DoH 1993).

Even when women do have a clear preference, the maternity service may be unable or unwilling to help women achieve that choice. In the 1960s women who wanted hospital births were not always able to obtain them. Now, in spite of a change in policy, there is considerable anecdotal and some survey evidence that women are not able to obtain home births. A survey of 253 women residing in the former Northern Regional Health Authority area in England who had expressed a wish to give birth at home found that 14 per cent of these women were actively dissuaded by those caring for them from having a home birth, but not for any obstetric reason (Davies *et al* 1996). The view that women are often put off choosing a home birth by their GP has been given greater credence by a postal survey of GPs in West Sussex. This found that 'the majority felt that too much encouragement was being given for women to have their babies at home', and while most said they would be willing to continue to care for a woman who expressed a wish for a home birth, 5 per cent indicated that they would in such circumstances remove the woman from their list (Higson 1996).

■ Costs

The Expert Maternity Group set as an objective for *Changing childbirth* that 'The service provided must represent value for money and the cost and benefit of alternative arrangements [be] assessed locally'. Interestingly, the Expert Maternity Group did not itself cost the proposals it was making. This may, in part, be a reflection of the paucity of information on the comparative costs of providing maternity care in different settings.

In the past, small obstetric units and isolated GP units were closed on the basis that they were not as cost effective as large centralised consultant obstetric units. What little evidence there is dates mostly from the 1970s and tends to point to the opposite conclusion. Moreover, as Mugford (1990) has pointed out, cost effectiveness is 'a relative concept, and requires comparative evidence about the cost effectiveness of consultant obstetric care. This has yet to be studied in any detail.'

A study comparing the average costs of maternity care in consultant units and GP units in one health board in Scotland found the cost of consultant unit care to be higher, particularly on the day of delivery. However, no allowance was made in the analysis for differences in the types of delivery being undertaken (Gray & Steel 1981). Ferster and Pethybridge (1973) undertook a comparison of the costs of providing maternity care in a consultant unit, in an urban GP unit, as an urban home delivery, as delivery in four rural GP units and as rural home delivery. By separating out births in which there was intervention at delivery, some adjustment for case mix was made. The costs of GP services and those of the local authorities who at that time paid for community midwives were taken into account, but the costs to families were not. Costs in all four of the isolated GP units were found to be high whether or not there was intervention, but costs in the urban unit were generally much less. Costs in the consultant unit were also high if there was intervention during delivery but otherwise were low. The cost of home delivery was lower, particularly in rural areas.

In the only study to take account of family costs, the cost for women who had booked for delivery at home were compared with those of a matched group of women booked for birth in a GP unit. This was in turn compared with estimates of the cost of a normal delivery in a consultant unit. Consultant unit delivery was found to be the most expensive, both to the public purse and to the family. Home delivery was the least expensive form of care as far as public sector costs were concerned, but family costs were at their lowest when the delivery took place in a GP unit (Stilwell 1979).

Unlike the Expert Maternity Group, the Scottish Home and Health Department's review of maternity services did provide estimates of the cost of providing maternity care in different places (SHHD 1993). Details of these are given in Table 1.3. These estimates were based on the original place of booking and therefore include the cost of transfer. In these circumstances, the average cost of delivery outside a consultant unit will vary considerably, depending what assumptions are made about transfer rates. As has been noted elsewhere in this chapter, the empirical evidence is that there are substantial differences in transfer rates.

Table 1.3 Estimated costs of providing maternity care in different settings in Scotland according to the original place of booking

Consultant unit	
Low risk	£1661
High risk	£2535
GP maternity unit	£1991
Domino delivery	£1446
Home delivery	£1407

Data from Scottish Home and Health Department, 1993.

The idea that small maternity units are 'not economic to run' can be traced back to economic theory suggesting that, as organizations grow, they become more efficient in their use of resources because fixed costs (examples in maternity care would include the cost of maintenance of buildings or providing senior medical and midwifery staff) are spread over a larger number of units of output (in this context, women delivering babies). This is often referred to as achieving 'economies of scale'.

The extent to which this theoretical principle operates in practice in the health service has been called into question (Mugford 1990). Using DHSS costing returns for the financial year 1985/86, Mugford has shown that patient care costs actually rise as hospital size increases, probably because more serious cases are treated in larger hospitals. Moreover, her findings show that the general costs of running hospitals do not vary according to the size of the hospital.

Evidence on the costs of providing different types of maternity care in different places is still very patchy. What does exist does not seem to support the conventional wisdom that centralising care in large obstetric units will reduce costs.

■ Conclusions

After a long and very detailed review of all the scientific evidence available for the UK, the key elements of which have been summarised in this chapter, it was concluded (Campbell & Macfarlane 1994) that:

- There is no evidence to support the claim that the safest policy is for all women to give birth in hospital.

- The statistical association between the increase in the proportion of hospital deliveries and the fall in the crude perinatal mortality rate seems unlikely to be explained either wholly or in part by a cause and effect relationship.

- No satisfactory explanation has been found for the higher crude perinatal mortality rate observed for births occurring before the mid 1970s in hospitals with consultant obstetric facilities compared with those in other places.

- Lack of data means that it is not possible to conclude, with any degree of confidence, that babies born to low risk women in hospitals with consultant obstetric facilities are exposed to a greater or lesser risk of death due to obstetric intervention than similar babies born elsewhere.

- The rise between 1970 and 1980 in the crude perinatal mortality rate for births at home can almost certainly be explained by the disproportionate increase in the proportion of unplanned births at home relative to those planned to occur there, as a consequence of the fall in the overall number of home births.

- The policy of closing small obstetric units on the grounds of safety or cost is not supported by the available evidence.

- For women at low risk who give birth in hospital, there is no clear evidence of differences between the mortality and morbidity of babies born to women giving birth under the care of consultant obstetricians and those whose deliveries are supervised by general practitioners.

- The poorer outcomes among women transferred from home or general practitioner units compared with women who were not transferred probably result from selective referral of women with problems. Although there is no conclusive evidence, it is likely that this selection process, rather than the adverse effects of obstetric intervention, accounts for high mortality rates in hospital, compared with planned births at home or in isolated general practitioner units.

- There is some evidence, although not conclusive, that morbidity is higher among mothers and babies cared for in an institutional setting. For some women, it is possible, but not proven, that the iatrogenic risk associated with institutional delivery may be greater than any benefit conferred.

- The few studies of cost done in the United Kingdom have found no evidence that care in general practitioner maternity units is uneconomic for the public sector or its users. There is insufficient recent evidence from which to draw any conclusions about the cost of home births.

- A majority of women who had experienced both home and hospital deliveries preferred to have their babies at home, although they are more likely to include a disproportionate number of women who had sought home delivery after a hospital delivery with which they had been dissatisfied.

■ Recommendations for clinical practice in the light of currently available evidence

1. 'Women should receive clear, unbiased advice and be able to choose where they would like their baby to be born. Their right to make that choice should be respected and every practical effort made to achieve the outcome that the woman believes is best for her baby and herself' (DoH 1993).

2. It should not be assumed that women want a hospital birth because they have not explicitly stated a preference for something else. Women

need to be given time to consider the options available and be able to make an active choice.

3. Women need to be made aware that the place booked for delivery can change. They may wish to change their booking for non-medical reasons or because obstetric complications develop and the outcome is likely to be improved if the delivery takes place in hospital.

4. If a change of booking or transfer in labour is made for obstetric reasons, this should be fully discussed with the woman. Where possible, the midwife transferring a woman into hospital during labour should remain involved in her care, if that is what the woman wants.

5. When a woman booked for delivery outside a consultant obstetric unit is referred to an obstetrician because of the development of complications, she should be referred back to the original place of booking if the complication resolves. At present, transfer of booking mostly appears to take place in one direction.

6. If professionals caring for a pregnant woman think that a birth outside a consultant obstetric unit poses a particular risk to a woman and/or her baby, the precise nature of the risk should be explained to the woman. Where possible, this advice should be based on reliable research evidence.

■ Practice check

-   What are your own beliefs about the comparative safety of home and hospital birth? Have they changed in the light of the information contained in this chapter?

-   What information would you give to a woman who asks about a home birth?

-   What do you currently tell women about the alternatives available to them?

-   How many home births have you attended? If you have not had recent experience of a home delivery, could you rectify this?

-   Consider your own skills regarding the critical appraisal of research literature so that not every report is accepted unquestioningly.

☐ Acknowledgements

The author wishes to thank Alison Macfarlane of the National Perinatal Epidemiology Unit, Oxford, co-author of *Where to be born? The debate and the evidence*, from which parts of this chapter have been drawn.

■ References

Allison J 1996 Delivered at home. Chapman & Hall, London

Alment EAJ, Barr A, Reid M *et al* 1967 Normal confinement: a domiciliary and hospital study. British Medical Journal 2: 530–5

Ashford JR 1978 Policies for maternity care in England and Wales: too fast and too far? In Kitzinger S, Davis JA (eds) The place of birth. Oxford University Press, Oxford, Ch 2

Ayres R 1996 Midwife led care working alongside a GP service: the Exeter experience. Paper presented at Changing Childbirth Regional Conference, Weston-Super-Mare, March

Barron SL, Thomson AM, Philips PR 1977 Home and hospital confinement in Newcastle-upon-Tyne 1960–69. British Journal of Obstetrics and Gynaecology 84: 401–11

Black N 1982 Do general practitioner deliveries constitute a perinatal mortality risk? British Medical Journal 284: 488–90

Campbell R 1990 The place of birth. In Alexander J, Levy V, Roch S (eds) Intrapartum care: a research-based approach. Macmillan, Basingstoke, Ch 1

Campbell R, Macfarlane AJ 1990 General practitioner maternity units. British Medical Journal 301: 983–4 (letter)

Campbell R, Macfarlane A 1994 Where to be born? The debate and the evidence, 2nd edn. National Perinatal Epidemiology Unit, Oxford

Campbell R, Macfarlane A 1996 Evaluation of the midwife-led unit at the Royal Bournemouth Hospital. Unpublished study

Campbell R, Macdonald Davies I, Macfarlane AJ *et al* 1984 Home births in England and Wales; perinatal mortality according to intended place of delivery. British Medical Journal 289: 721–4

Chalmers I, Zlosnik JE, Johns KA *et al* 1976 Obstetric practice and outcome of pregnancy in Cardiff residents 1965–1973. British Medical Journal i: 735–8

Chamberlain G, Philipp E, Hewlett B *et al* 1978 British births 1970, vol. 2, Obstetric care. Heinemann, London

Charney M 1990 General practitioner maternity units. British Medical Journal 301: 664–5 (letter)

Clarke M, Mason ES, MacVicar J *et al* 1993 Evaluating perinatal mortality rates: effects of referral and case mix. British Medical Journal 306: 824–7

Creasy JM 1994 Women's experience of transfer from community based to consultant care in late pregnancy or labour. MPhil thesis, Department of General Practice, Sheffield University

Davies J, Hey E, Reid W, Young G 1996 Prospective regional study of planned home births. British Medical Journal 313: 1302–6

Department of Health 1993 Changing childbirth, part I. Report of the Expert Maternity Group. HMSO, London

Donnison J 1977 Midwives and medical men. Schocken Books, New York

Dowswell T, Thornton JG, Hewison J, Lilford RJL 1996 Should there be a trial of home versus hospital delivery in the United Kingdom? British Medical Journal 313: 753

Ferster G, Pethybridge R 1973 The cost of a local maternity care system. Hospital and Health Services Review July: 243–7

Fleury PM 1967 Maternity care. Mothers' experience of childbirth. Allen & Unwin, London

Fryer JG, Ashford A 1972 Trends in perinatal and neonatal mortality in England and Wales 1960–69. British Journal of Preventative and Social Medicine 26: 1–9

Garrett T, House W, Lowe SW 1987 Outcome of women booked into an isolated general practice maternity unit over eight years. Journal of the Royal College of General Practitioners 37: 488–90

Golding J, Peters T 1988 Are hospital confinements really bad for the fetus? Early Human Development 17: 29–36

Goldthorp WO, Richman J 1974 Maternal attitudes to unintended home confinement. A case study of the effects of the hospital strike upon domiciliary confinements. Practitioner 212: 845–53

Gordon I, Elias-Jones TF 1960 The place of confinement: home or hospital? The mother's preference. British Medical Journal 1: 52–3

Gray AM, Steele R 1981 The economics of specialist and general practitioner maternity units. Journal of the Royal College of General Practitioners 31: 586–92

Green JM, Coupland VA, Kitzinger JV et al 1988 Great expectations: a prospective study of women's expectations and experiences of childbirth. Child Care Development Groups, University of Cambridge

Higson N 1996 GPs lack information about Changing Childbirth. Changing Childbirth Update 6: 11

Hobbs MST, Acheson ED 1966a Obstetric care in the first pregnancy. Lancet i: 761–4

Hobbs MST, Acheson ED 1966b Perinatal mortality and the organisation of obstetric services in the Oxford area in 1962. British Medical Journal 1: 499

House of Commons 1985 Official report Session 1984–85. Reply to a written question by John Patten. Hansard 70: 878–84

House of Commons 1987 Written reply by Mrs Currie. Hansard Nov 6: col 919

House of Commons Health Committee 1992 Maternity services. vol. I (Chairman N Winterton). HC 29–I. HMSO, London.

Hudson CK 1968 Domiciliary obstetrics in a group practice. Practitioner 201: 816–22

Hundley VA, Cruickshank FM, Lang GD et al 1994 Midwife managed delivery unit: randomised controlled comparison with consultant-led care. British Medical Journal 309: 1400–4

Hundley VA, Cruickshank FM, Milne J et al 1995 Costs of intrapartum care in a midwife managed delivery unit and a consultant led labour ward. Midwifery 11: 103–9

Jackson K 1996 Changing maternity services across national boundaries. Changing Childbirth across nations. Keynote address at the International Congress of Midwifery, Oslo, May

Jacoby A, Cartwright A 1990 Finding out about the views and experiences of maternity service users. In Garcia J, Kilpatrick R, Richards M (eds) The politics of maternity care. Oxford University Press, Oxford, Ch 13

Jarvis SN, Holloway JS, Hey E 1985 Increase in cerebral palsy in normal birthweight babies. Archives of Disease in Childhood 60: 1113–21

Johnson M, Smith J, Haddad S et al 1992 Women prefer hospital births. British Medical Journal 305: 255 (letter)

Klein M, Lloyd I, Redman C et al 1983 A comparison of low-risk pregnant women booked for delivery in two systems of care: shared care (consultant) and integrated general practice unit. British Journal of Obstetrics and Gynaecology 99: 118–22

Lilford RJ 1987 Clinical experimentation in obstretrics. British Medical Journal 295: 1298–1300

Local Government Board 1918 Forty-seventh annual report of the Local Government Board, 1917–18, part I. Cmnd 9157. HMSO, London

Lowe SW, House W, Garrett T 1987 Comparison of outcome of low risk labour in an isolated general practice maternity unit and a specialist maternity hospital. Journal of the Royal College of General Practitioners 37: 484–7

Macfarlane M, Mugford M, Johnson A, Garcia J 1995 Counting the changes in childbirth: trends and gaps in national statistics. National Perinatal Epidemiology Unit, Oxford

MacVicar J, Dobbie G, Owen-Johnstone L, Jagger C, Hopkins M, Kennedy J 1993 Simulated home delivery in hospital: a randomised controlled trial. British Journal of Obstetrics and Gynaecology   100: 316–23

Mason V 1990 Women's experience of maternity care – a survey manual. HMSO, London

Maternity Services Advisory Committee 1984 Maternity care in action, part II, Care during childbirth (intrapartum care); a guide to good practice and a plan for action. HMSO, London

Ministry of Health 1959 Report of the Maternity Services Committee (Chairman Lord Cranbrook). HMSO, London

Mugford M 1990 Economies of scale in low risk maternity care: what is the evidence? Maternity Action   46: 6–8

Northern Regional Perinatal Mortality Survey Coordinating Group 1996 Collaborative survey of perinatal loss in planned and unplanned home births. British Medical Journal   313: 1306–9

O'Brien M 1978 Home and hospital confinement: a comparison of the experiences of mothers having home and hospital confinements. Journal of the Royal College of General Practitioners   28: 460–6

Peretz EA 1990 Maternity service for England and Wales: local authority maternity care in the inter-war period in Oxfordshire and Tottenham. In Garcia J, Kilpatrick R, Richards M (eds) The politics of maternity care. Oxford University Press, Oxford, Ch 2

Prentice A, Walton SM 1989 Outcome of pregnancies referred to a general practitioner maternity unit in a district general hospital. British Medical Journal   299: 1090–2

President of the Royal College of Obstetricians and Gynaecologists, President of the Royal College of Midwives, Chairman of the Royal College of General Practitioners 1992 Maternity care in the new NHS. A joint approach. RCOG, RCM, RCGP, London

Reynolds JL, Yudkin PL, Bull MJV 1988 General practitioner obstetrics: does risk prediction work? Journal of the Royal College of General Practitioners   38: 307–10

Royal College of Midwives 1987 Towards a healthy nation. RCM, London

Royal College of Obstetricians and Gynaecologists 1944 Report on a national maternity service. RCOG, London

Royal College of Obstetricians and Gynaecologists 1954 Report on the obstetric service under the NHS. RCOG, London

Rutter P 1964 Domiciliary midwifery: is it justifiable? Lancet   ii: 1228–30

Sangala V, Dunster G, Bohin S, Osbourne JP 1990 Perinatal mortality rates in isolated general practitioner maternity units. British Medical Journal   301: 418–20

Scottish Office Home and Health Department 1993 Provision of maternity services in Scotland. A policy review. HMSO, Edinburgh

Shearer JML 1985 Five year prospective survey of risk of booking for a home birth. British Medical Journal   291: 1478–80

Smith FB 1979 The people's health 1830–1910. Croom Helm, London

Social Services Committee 1980 Perinatal and neonatal mortality. Second report from the Social Services Committee, Session 1979–80, vol. I (Chairman R Short). HC 663–I. HMSO, London

Standing Maternity and Midwifery Advisory Committee 1970 Domiciliary midwifery and maternity bed needs (Chairman J Peel). HMSO, London

Stilwell JA 1979 Relative costs of home and hospital confinements. British Medical Journal   2: 257–9

Taylor A 1986 Maternity services: the consumer's view. Journal of the Royal College of General Practitioners   36: 157–60

Taylor GW, Edgar W, Taylor BA, Neal DG 1980 How safe is general practitioner obstetrics? Lancet   ii: 1287–9

Tew M 1978 The case against hospital deliveries: the statistical evidence. In Kitzinger S, Davis JA (eds) The place of birth. Oxford University Press, Oxford, Ch 4

Tew M 1981 Effects of scientific obstetrics on perinatal mortality. Health Services Journal   91: 444–6

Tew M 1986 Do obstetric intranatal interventions make birth safer? British Journal of Obstetrics and Gynaecology   93: 659–74

Tew M 1990 Safer childbirth? Chapman & Hall, London

Turnbull D, Holmes A, Shields N *et al* 1996 Randomised, controlled trial of efficacy of midwife-managed care. Lancet   348: 213–18

Woodall J 1968 No place like home. Proceedings of the Royal Society of Medicine 61: 1032–4

Young G 1987 Are isolated maternity units run by general practitioners dangerous? British Medical Journal   294: 744–6

Zander L, Klein M 1989 Role of the family practitioner in maternity care. In Chalmers I, Enkin M, Keirse MJNC (eds) Effective care in pregnancy and childbirth. Oxford University Press, Oxford, Ch 11

Chapter 2

Motherhood as a rite of passage: an anthropological perspective

Carole Yearley

For many women, becoming a mother means changes to their lives that are often unimaginable until they have experienced motherhood for themselves. Women describe intense feelings associated with motherhood, ranging from overwhelming love to resentment towards their babies (Ball 1989), and Holden (1990) argues that the depth of these emotions sometimes surprises and dismays the women themselves.

Pregnancy and childbirth are normal physiological processes, yet the latter is an event that is full of ritual and cultural meanings that vary extensively from society to society. As Kitzinger (1978: 105) argues, human pregnancy and childbirth are cultural acts in which 'Spontaneous physiological processes operate within a context of customs'. It is the cultural context in which maternity is set that dictates the way in which these physiological events are perceived and the responses they initiate.

The aim of this chapter is to offer an anthropological perspective of birth as a cultural event. It will demonstrate that birth is an occasion that utilises rituals associated with pregnancy, childbirth and becoming a mother. Examples from different societies will be used to illustrate the cultural diversity of pregnancy and childbirth and how women make the transition from one social status to another. It will be argued that the erosion of some of these important rites of passage may adversely affect the way in which women from Western, industrialised societies negotiate and adapt to their new role as mothers. The chapter, by encouraging midwives to become aware of the cultural needs of their clients, attempts to address some of the negative emotions and unhappiness that appear to affect so many new mothers in Britain. It is anticipated that a deeper understanding of these issues will enable midwives to adopt strategies for practice that will help their clients towards a smoother transition to motherhood.

■ It is assumed that you are already aware of the following:

- The physiological and psychological changes that occur following childbirth;

- The midwife's responsibilities and sphere of practice in relation to the provision of postnatal care to mothers and babies (UKCC 1993);

- The diversity of the client group for the area in which you practise, including the range of ethnic and social backgrounds.

■ The meaning and importance of culture

Cultural values associated with childbirth and motherhood underpin the adaptation of women to their new social status and the way in which they are perceived and responded to by society. Helman (1990) describes culture as a set of explicit and implicit guidelines that individuals inherit as members of a particular society. He asserts that these inform group members about how to view their world, how to experience it emotionally, and how to behave within it in response to other people, to nature and to supernatural forces. Moreover, culture enables the members to transmit these guidelines to the next generation by the use of symbols, language, art and ritual. Helman (1990: 3) likens culture to an 'inherited lens' through which 'individuals perceive and understand the world that they inhabit and learn how to live within it'. Culture is acquired almost unnoticed, as a result of an individual growing up within a given society and gradually acquiring the unique cultural 'lens' of that society. Helman (1990: 3) concludes that, without the shared perception of the world, the 'cohesion and continuity of any human group would be impossible'. Although 'culture' is often talked about as if it is something that affects others, particularly those from exotic backgrounds, cultural values are intrinsically woven into the very fabric of every known society, including, of course, our own.

Midwives come into contact with a diverse range of people, each one of whose values and beliefs are shaped by the culture of the society in which they live. This too applies to the midwife, who is likewise a member of a group and is thus also culturally influenced. The midwife needs to develop skills of self-awareness in order to recognise that her personal value system may differ from that of her client; some differences are more obvious than others. The midwife also needs to be critical of texts offering a mere 'laundry list' of the cultural behaviours of different ethnic groups. Culture is dynamic, and not all Pakistani or Jewish women, for example, will be totally traditional; people learn their culture as opposed to being taught it. Therefore ethnically sensitive practice and care have to emerge from discussions between midwives and women, without expectations being imposed on clients simply because such behaviour is assumed by the midwife to be the 'norm' for a particular ethnic group. Such skills will enable midwives to acquire a deeper understanding of the different ways in which women, their partners and their families respond to and negotiate the transition into motherhood. Knowledge of the client's belief systems will contribute towards providing the kind of maternity care that is appropriate, acceptable and offered in a way that respects a woman's cultural values.

■ Social transition, liminality and motherhood

Pregnancy and childbirth are a unique journey for each woman, during which she transcends one social status to achieve another. Van Gennep (1960) identified three phases of this processual form:

1. The rites of separation, often accompanied by rituals and symbolic behaviour, which separate the individual (both privately and publicly) from his or her former social state;

2. Liminal rites, which signify the person's temporary marginality;

3. The reincorporation of the individual back into society, often with an altered social status.

These phases do not always remain discrete but may merge one into another. Collectively, Van Gennep referred to the phases as the 'rites of passage'.

Turner (1974) argues that it is the liminal phase or the 'betwixt and between' phase of the two social states that is fraught with both danger and opportunity. It is this separation from existing social structures into liminality which Turner refers to as 'communitas', a condition on the peripheries of everyday life during which the individual undergoes some personal transformation. Many traditional societies themselves view pregnancy and childbirth as events that place the woman in a state of liminality (Faithorn 1975; Okeley 1977; Homans 1982). Her status changes from 'wife' to 'mother' during the course of the transition and places her in a temporary state of 'limbo'. During this time, she may be considered to be in an ambiguous and socially abnormal situation, vulnerable to outside dangers and sometimes to others because she has departed from the safety of her old status but not yet established herself within her new one.

Jeffery and Jeffery (1993), in their ethnographic study of women and childbearing in rural Bijnor, Northern India, maintain that the community perceives death to be a threat that is greatest around the time of birth. Death itself is considered taboo as it presents a danger to others from its polluting effects. In traditional societies, such as that of Bijnor, maternal mortality is known and recognised to be a common event. The blood of childbirth and the ensuing lochia are considered to be highly polluting since they are particularly alluring to evil spirits. The woman's liminal state is therefore maintained until the cessation of her lochia. She is often segregated and isolated from the rest of the community, apart from one or two elderly female carers, in order to protect others and herself from her dangerous state. Tasks such as cooking are forbidden lest she contaminates the family's food, and worship is prohibited because of the shamefulness of her condition (Jeffery *et al* 1989).

Pregnancy in rural Bijnor is perceived as a shameful and defiling event. It demonstrates a woman's sexuality and is therefore, as far as possible, concealed and ignored by others in the community. Jeffery *et al* (1989) found that antenatal care was virtually non-existent for these women and perceived by them to be a luxury afforded only to the rich. Pregnancy does not permit exemption from the daily grind of chores for the young married women (bahus) as they make up an important part of the labour force, frequently having to continue with strenuous manual work right up to, and even during, the early stages of labour. This is in contrast to the care for Western women, who are encouraged to avoid activities such as heavy lifting and to take maternity leave from paid employment during pregnancy.

Pregnancy in Western industrialised societies such as Britain, on the other hand, is a relatively public affair, which is accorded a high media and consumer profile. For example, a lucrative fashion industry has developed which responds to consumer demands for clothes that acknowledge and flatter the pregnant body. British women also have access to a wide variety of literature, which, although set within a medical framework, offers information and advises on all aspects of pregnancy and childbirth as well as on how to prepare for and act in the new role as a mother. Antenatal care and parenthood education are available to all and are seen and used by the majority as a sound investment towards a successful outcome of pregnancy.

In a society such as Bijnor, where pregnancy is not acknowledged because of its shameful nature, young pregnant bahus have no such access to information or advice. Once married, they leave the villages where they were born and frequently travel a great distance in order to live with their husbands' kin. They have no-one with whom they can discuss the physical and psychological changes they may be experiencing, and Jeffery and Jeffery (1993) maintain that the women in their study enjoyed less social and emotional support during pregnancy and childbirth than anthropologists suggest is afforded to pregnant women in other cultures.

☐ Summary

Pregnancy and childbirth are marked by contrasting rites of separation from the woman's existing role and status, which are dependent upon the social context in which pregnancy is set. At one extreme, women may experience an increasing sense of isolation during pregnancy, because of the obvious evidence of their sexuality, while for other women pregnancy and childbirth are a matter of public interest and concern.

■ The significance of ritual

The liminal states of pregnancy and childbirth are marked with rituals, which fulfil an important role for the woman and society as they formally recognise and acknowledge her altering status. Loudon (1966) asserts that rituals are a feature common to all human societies and describes them as including prescribed and repetitive formal behaviours, which have no obvious technical consequences but which are symbolic in nature. Helman (1990) argues that this implies that the behaviour or actions say something about the state of affairs, both in society and at large, and on the social conditions of the performers of the ritual in particular.

Rituals that mark the changing status of women during pregnancy in non-industrialised societies sometimes appear bizarre when viewed from the perspective of one living outside that particular society. However, practices are also commonly adopted in the West which are ritualistic, serving little or no technical purpose save to signify the altering status of the woman. Examples include the routine weighing of women during the antenatal period (Hytten 1980) and other procedures that are adhered to on admission of women to the labour ward. These formerly included practices such as the routine perineal shave and enema. More recently, the donning of a hospital gown on admission serves to represent that the woman has entered an institution, thus agreeing, albeit subconsciously, to accept and condone those procedures and policies associated with the dominant institution of the hospital (Turner 1990).

The Expert Maternity Group (DoH 1993) emphasises the importance of individualised, woman-centred maternity care. The implementation of the report's recommendations may challenge many of the accepted rituals that are incorporated within the provision of maternity care, for example the frequency and pattern of antenatal visits, which has been in place for nearly a century, and the traditional 6-week postnatal check-up. Some rituals are, in fact, not solely symbolic, in that they sometimes produce negative outcomes for women and their babies.

Rituals are intrinsic to any transition, and Turner (1982) identified two functions of rituals. First, they symbolically express certain fundamental values and cultural orientations through the use of dramatic performance. According to Frankenberg (1986), dramatic performance is a mode of human behaviour or an approach to experience. It is a play and much more, and the consequences of human interaction in terms of performance and drama help us to understand the impact that social processes have on the meaning of certain life events such as childbirth. Second, such dramas communicate key values to all those involved, and the use of symbols is necessary in achieving the expression and communication of ritual. Examples of some symbols of rituals could be the doctor's white coat and stethoscope.

Homans (1982) concludes that all pregnant women, regardless of social class and ethnic background, observe some rituals during pregnancy. She argues that, during the transition from pregnancy to motherhood, women face periods of uncertainty and have both specific and nameless fears. The adoption of rituals may help to signify and ease their transition, but health carers must guard against the use of practices that may produce negative outcomes for their clients, ensuring that their practice is research based and sensitive to the individual needs of the woman.

Over the past two decades, there has been a growing body of valuable research into midwifery, undertaken by midwives and associated health carers, with the aim of improving the quality of care in the maternity services. While these innovations are exciting, an anthropological focus in midwifery research may further extend our understanding of the ways in which culture modifies and influences women's experiences of pregnancy and childbirth. Doughtery and Tripp-Reimer (1990) have recognised that parallels can be drawn between the disciplines of anthropology and nursing. It would appear there is even greater potential for the application of anthropology to midwifery because of the cultural diversity associated with pregnancy and childbirth. The indications are that there is a need for further innovative research encompassing both midwifery and anthropology in order to expand our existing body of knowledge for the benefit of clients.

■ The emergence of the new mother

Van Gennep (1960) argues that, in the final phase of motherhood as a rite of passage, the physiological 'return' is secondary to the social 'return' from childbirth. Following the birth, it is common in many traditional societies for the woman to observe a period of withdrawal from the community. Homans (1982) reported that the length of seclusion in India varied from 10 days for women in the highest caste (the Brahmins) to 40 days among those in the lower castes. Traditionally, the woman and her baby are expected to remain confined during this period, and she is exempt from her normal duties. Care is provided by other female relatives, most commonly the mother-in-law, the mother's time being spent exclusively attending to, and breastfeeding, her new baby.

Traditionally, postpartum restrictions were also observed for women in Britain, although they appear to have lost much of their significance nowadays, sometimes to the detriment of new mothers. In past decades, it was commonly expected that mothers in Britian would observe a 10-day 'lying-in' period following delivery. On completion of this, they would return to their homes, emerging into their new role and position in society (Helman 1990). Homans (1982) recalls a ceremony of significance in Britain, namely the 'churching of women'. This involved worship by the mother and her community whereby thanks were offered to God for delivering the mother from the 'great pain and peril of childbirth', to quote the *Book of Common Prayer* (Batchelor 1980). It also signified the end of the liminal phase of transition, marking her final cleansing from potential pollution prior to her re-integration into society within her new social status. This ceremony presented an opportunity for celebration as the woman was formally welcomed back into her community and congratulated by her family and friends.

The most common ceremonies still practised are the christening and circumcision rituals, which focus primarily on the baby's incorporation into religious and social life rather than on the mother. Pillsbury (1978) argues that it is the attention and support of the social network in the first few weeks following the birth that help the mother to adjust to her new role in society.

This is in contrast to the experiences of many new mothers in Britain today who return home to relative isolation. The advent of industrialisation has displaced the home from being the central locus of productivity (Price & Bamford 1974; Giddens 1989) and irrevocably altered many of the traditional features of the pre-industrial era, such as the extended family. Couples move great distances from their parents, siblings and friends, with whom they grew up, in pursuit of work and career opportunities. Work-based activities that keep women away from their new homes may mean that they lack the local support from family and friends that would have been taken for granted in their own mothers' and grandmothers' days.

Midwives are in an optimal position to offer practical help that could reduce the isolation that some women experience following childbirth. Flint (1986) identifies recommendations that can be easily and inexpensively incorporated into practice, which, with a little innovative thought and planning, can help to build support networks with other local mothers. The midwife may consider herself as a facilitator, one who initiates contacts between women in her care. She can help friendships to develop antenatally through parenthood education classes and enable these women to keep in touch postnatally. In this way, new mothers can experience the transition together, receiving continuing support and friendship from each other long after they have been discharged from the midwife's care.

■ Transition and role conflict

Oakley (1980) writes that women have to undergo the greatest adaptation following the birth of their first baby, and Hall (1987) concludes that first time mothers perceive their transition to motherhood as being one that incorporates a process of role redefinition. Although Hall's study focuses primarily on the experiences of first time mothers returning to the workplace, her work is relevant as the three stages she identified can be applied as a model for all women undergoing the transition to motherhood, particularly for the first time. According to Hall (1987), the stages are: taking on multiple roles, experiencing role strain and reducing role strain.

A wide variation in gender cultures exists throughout the world, and what is seen as typical behaviour for women in a given society may not be regarded as such in another. For example, women in many Islamic cultures are restricted to the home and undertake solely domestic roles, such as childcare and running the home (Ember & Ember 1985). In other traditional societies, Helman (1990) argues that, in addition to maintaining their domestic role, women are also involved in raising the livestock and in the planting, cultivation and harvesting of crops, as well as in the production of clothes, pottery and handicrafts for sale at market. In industrialised societies such as northern Europe, Ember and Ember (1985) reported that over 50 per cent of women worked outside the home, a figure that is surely considerably higher today. Women from both traditional and industrialised societies undertake multiple roles, which may cause stress when their personal resources are stretched, prompting them to seek ways in which to reduce this strain.

Hall's model of role redefinition (1987) has the potential for use by midwives and may help them to anticipate and reduce the difficulties that some women encounter in their transition to motherhood. If the midwife is to provide the appropriate kind of help and support, however, it is vital that she appreciates that the role redefinition process changes as the mother passes through and negotiates her personal transition through the various stages of the childbearing process. The preconceptual, antenatal, and early and late postnatal phases complete the transition from woman to mother.

Women can only imagine how motherhood will influence them before it becomes reality. Any decisions made are intuitive ones, although research indicates that some women do make choices relating to specific issues, such as infant feeding and resuming employment, prior to becoming mothers (Oakley 1979; Hall 1987; Thomson 1989). Midwives could take more positive steps to encourage women to make informed decisions rather than just intuitive ones in order to ease their transition to motherhood. Women need to be encouraged to approach motherhood with realistic expectations. Opportunities could be made for open discussion of the feelings and expectations of women, their partners and others who matter in their lives. In this way, couples and their families could anticipate how they might identify for themselves personal role strain, the factors causing it, and how to take positive steps to reduce it. The outcome in terms of promoting the health and wellbeing of the new mother and enhancing family stability could have positive effects on the whole society.

Many mothers in the industrialised West experience role conflict, receiving opposing messages from society about what a 'good mother' should be. Dally (1982) argues that the media and society idealise motherhood, yet they undervalue the home-centred mother. Motherhood is perceived as a highly valued goal in many societies, which increases a woman's status and elevates her social position, earning her greater respect within her community (Boddy 1989). Indeed, in Sri Lanka, McGilvray (1982) found that if a woman cannot bear a child, she is apportioned the blame for the infertility and may be abandoned in favour of one who can become pregnant (Laderman 1983). Infertility in the West is also taboo, yet motherhood is not highly prized (Dally 1982), and some women find that, in terms of employment opportunities and finance, they are in fact penalised by society for becoming mothers.

Social and political messages persist that the mother's role should be one of dutiful passivity. Palmer (1988) argues that, in the workplace, women who return to work after having a baby are frequently exploited, taking jobs that fit in around the family rather than being in accordance with their training or talents (Steiner 1989). However, motherhood is in many cultures respected as an 'occupation' (MacCormack 1982), and children are regarded as the hope for the future, thus being considered as the community's greatest resource.

Pregnancy and childbirth in the West are generally regarded as being legally in the public domain. Pregnant women are recognised by society as being in a special situation and are thus entitled to certain rights in terms of financial and maternity health care. Yet many of these privileges are withdrawn soon after childbirth, and mothers are encouraged to resume their combined social roles of mother, wife and lover as soon as possible. Kruckman (1992) argues that initiatives intended to improve maternity care, such as encouraging an early transfer home from hospital, may potentially reduce the time for women to adjust to motherhood, and the outcome of these initiatives may result in a social and public policy that fails to recognise the woman's change in status. The lack of clear role redefiniton and the inadequate provision of social support deny many women the rites of passage necessary to facilitate their transition into motherhood. It appears that such denial contributes significantly to the unhappiness that many women experience after childbirth within modern industrialised societies (Stern & Kruckman 1983).

■ The impact of the political economy on the transition to motherhood

The rites of passage that mark the transition to motherhood are collectively shared by those within any given society and are set within its social context. While the experience of the transition itself is a personal one, it is influenced by the wider sociopolitical and economic forces of that society. Scheper-Hughes (1992) provides a moving ethnography of life in the poverty stricken shanty town of Alto do Cruzerio, northeast Brazil, where infant mortality is such a common feature of everyday life that even the mothers of the infants do not weep when their babies die. Rites of passage that signify the baby as a member of the community, such as the naming service and baptism, are delayed in comparison to those of other societies. Indeed, the child frequently remains unnamed until he reaches his first birthday. It appears that the liminal period for the Alto mothers is protracted compared with that of Western mothers, who overtly demonstrate signs of maternal attachment soon after, and frequently before, the birth of their babies (Klauss & Kennell 1976; Hyde 1986).

Scheper-Hughes (1992: 412) argues that the biomedical model of bonding that is the accepted norm in the West makes alternative maternal emotions seem 'unnatural... almost criminal'. She argues that maternal sentiments are shaped by the wider political agendas and goals of a particular society. In societies such as Britain, where infants are regarded as the sole responsibility of the nuclear family, maternal–infant attachments are encouraged. The technology of antenatal screening plays an important role in humanising the fetus/baby before birth. The use of ultrasound enables the mother to 'see' as well as feel her baby, and Reid (1990) observes that this serves as an initial introduction to her child as a living being, which helps to facilitate the attachment process. Rothman (1984) acknowledges that difficulties are experienced by women with regard to prenatal diagnosis as they endeavour to suspend their feelings of maternal attachment until they are certain that test results show that the fetus is 'normal'. Until this time, they manage their pregnancy in a state of 'suspended animation'.

This liminal phase of suspended animation can be applied to the Alto mothers. Maternal sentiments are withheld until the child can prove that he or she is capable of survival against the odds. As further emotional protection, the shanty town mothers are slow to anthropomorphise their infants with the recognition of certain characteristics, which individualise and personalise them as their own offspring, in case they should die. It appears that the Alto women arm themselves against disappointment and loss through the delayed process of maternal attachment that Scheper-Hughes (1992: 410) calls 'guarded, watchful waiting'. She concludes that Alto women display stoicism towards infant death, but they are, in fact, no different from Western mothers in their capacity to feel emotion. It is, however, the suppression of those emotions in response to covert political agendas that maintain the *status quo* of a situation that would be unacceptable in the West. Scheper-Hughes (1991) is critical of a state and its health service that appears to accept such a high incidence of child death without question, and calls for the appointment of 'socially conscious physicians who are able to engage with individuals about matters both biological and existential, as well as economic and political' (p 1146). Until people recognise that the macrostructures of individual societies exert subtle and persuasive influences on their members, the social and political indifference towards infant mortality in northeast Brazil and towards other disenfranchised groups will remain unchallenged. (For further reading on these issues, see Freire, 1970.)

To summarise, the emotions that women experience as they become mothers are personal but are unconsciously influenced by wider external factors determining what is considered to be acceptable behaviour in any given society. Their responses are acquired through the process of developing cultural knowledge. Midwives and other health carers need to become politically aware if they are to serve as advocates for mothers in order to enable them to adjust smoothly into their new role of motherhood. Education about the basic cultural rules that shape the behaviour of specific ethnic groups will deepen the understanding of midwives and enable them to improve the quality of their care in a way both appropriate for the woman's needs and respectful of her belief system.

■ Conclusion

Women, particularly first time mothers, undergo a tremendous adaptation during pregnancy and childbirth. The adaptation is a process marked with rituals and resulting in a personal transformation. Some mothers negotiate the process more easily than others, and for women who have little social support, the transition may be more difficult. Becoming a mother means that the woman has to undertake and adapt to new and multiple roles. In the industrialised West, women are expected to cope with a variety of roles – wage-earner, lover, wife, mother – and frequently to undertake two or more roles simultaneously. Motherhood in some non-industrialised societies affords respect, and the early days permit women the seclusion and the care from others needed to adjust to their new status. In others, wider politico-economic influences affect the 'production' of maternal emotions and the ways in which mothers respond to their infants.

It is the author's personal view that denial of the rites of passage, which recognise a woman's changing status, could be a significant contributory factor towards the unhappiness that is such a common feature of Western mothers. Midwives are in an ideal position to facilitate the woman's transition. They can emphasise the importance of the postnatal period as a special time for recovery and adaptation during which the mother should be nurtured and cherished.

The study of anthropology has the potential to offer valuable insights into maternity care and the needs of women and their families. The indications are that there is a need for further anthropological research, and educators need to recognise that anthropology has a valuable contribution to make.

■ Recommendations for clinical practice in the light of currently available evidence

1. Midwives need a greater awareness of the importance and dynamic impact of culture on individual beliefs and behaviour. Anthropology as a discipline could be incorporated into the midwifery curriculum to encourage the development of practitioners who can offer a more holistic approach to care.

2. Care should be offered in a respectful, non-judgemental way, so that rituals that mark the rites of passage are encouraged. Rituals known to have detrimental health effects, such as female genital mutilation, should be discouraged through the process of education.

3. Midwives can help women and their partners towards a smoother transition to motherhood by enabling them to approach the demands of motherhood with realistic expectations. Antenatal parenthood education can provide a forum for discussion in which feelings can be addressed. A list of contact names, addresses and babies' birthdates will encourage mothers to keep in contact with one another postnatally.

4. The midwife can emphasise the importance of the postnatal period for women as a special phase that requires time for adaptation to the woman's new role. Family and friends can be valuable in offering practical help that allows the mother time and space to adjust physically and emotionally to the new demands of motherhood. The community midwife needs to address the importance of the woman's psychological adaptation as well as her physical recovery. Community visits could be extended beyond 28 days for those women with few social reserves in order to offer ongoing support and friendship.

5. Women who may experience difficulties in adapting to and coping with their new role need to be identified at the initial booking interview so that potential problems can be identified early on and addressed. Effective communication between midwives and other members of the multidisciplinary team will facilitate prompt referral where necessary.

6. Midwives need to develop a greater political awareness to recognise the wider issues that influence society's perception of motherhood. Becoming active members of a professional trade union and participation in local pressure groups, such as the Breastfeeding Initiative, provide valuable opportunities of extending horizons so that midwifery can be represented at government level. This could benefit the maternity services and the women who use them.

■ Practice check

- Are you aware of the ethnic backgrounds of the women in the area in which you are practising?

- Do you understand the basic principles that are fundamental to the cultural beliefs of your client group?

- Do the antenatal preparation classes at your unit provide a forum for open discussion as well as providing specific parenting information?

- Examine your own practice. Could any of your practice be said to be ritualistic?

- During the postnatal examination, do you allow sufficient time to listen to how the mother feels as well as carrying out the physical examination?

- How do you assist new mothers to establish social networks?

- Consider your own attitudes towards women from differing ethnic backgrounds. How do you respond to rituals and behaviours that appear strange to you? Do you have respect for their wishes?

☐ Acknowledgments

My heartfelt thanks to Ronnie Frankenberg for his encouragement, advice and wise words to improve the structure and anthropological content of the text.

■ References

Ball J 1989 Postnatal care and adjustment to motherhood. In Robinson S, Thomson A (eds) Midwives, research and childbirth, vol. 1. Chapman & Hall, London, Ch 8

Batchelor M 1980 Book of common prayer. Lion Publishing, Hertfordshire

Boddy J 1989 Wombs and alien spirits: women, men and the Zar cult in Northern Sudan. University of Wisconsin Press, Madison

Dally A 1982 Inventing motherhood. The consequences of an ideal. Burnett Books, London

Department of Health 1993 Changing childbirth. Report of the Expert Maternity Group, HMSO, London

Dougherty M, Tripp-Reimer T 1990 Nursing and anthropology. In Thomas M, Sargent C (eds) Medical anthropology. Contemporary theory and method. Praeger, London, Ch 10

Ember C, Ember M 1985 Cultural anthropology. Prentice Hall, New Jersey

Faithorn E 1975 The concept of pollution among the Kafe of the Papua New Guinea Highlands. In Reiter R (ed.) Toward an anthropology of women. Monthly Review Press, New York

Flint C 1986 Sensitive midwifery. Heinemann, London

Frankenberg R 1986 Sickness as cultural performance: drama, trajectory and pilgrimage. Root metaphors and the making of social disease. International Journal of Health Services 16(4): 603–26

Freire P 1970 Pedagogy of the oppressed. Seabury, New York

Giddens A 1989 Sociology. Polity Press, London

Hall W 1987 The experience of women returning to work following the birth of their first child. Midwifery 3: 187–95

Helman C 1990 Culture, health and illness, 2nd edn. Wright, London

Holden J 1990 Emotional problems associated with childbirth. In Alexander J, Levy V, Roch S (eds) Postnatal care: a research-based approach. Macmillan, London, Ch 3

Homans H 1982 Pregnancy and birth as rites of passage for two groups of women in Britain. In MacCormack C (ed.) Ethnography of fertility and birth. Academic Press, London, Ch 9

Hyde B 1986 An interview study of pregnant women's attitudes to ultrasound scanning. Social Science and Medicine 22(5): 587–92

Hytten F 1980 Weight gain in pregnancy. In Hytten F, Chamberlain G (eds) Clinical physiology in obstetrics. Blackwell, Oxford

Jeffery R, Jeffery P 1993 Traditional birth attendants in rural North India: the social organization of childbearing. In Lindenbaum S, Lock M (eds) Knowledge, power and practice. The anthropology of everyday life. California, London, Ch 1

Jeffery P, Jeffery R, Lyon A 1989 Labour pains and labour power: women and child-bearing in India. Zed Books, London

Kitzinger S 1978 Women as mothers. Fontana, Glasgow

Klauss M, Kennell J 1976 Maternal–infant bonding. CV Mosby, St Louis.

Kruckman L 1992 Rituals and support: an anthropological view of postpartum depression. In Hamilton J, Harberger P (eds) Postpartum psychiatric illness. A picture puzzle. University of Pennsylvania Press, Philadelpia, Ch 11

Laderman C 1983 Childbirth and nutrition in rural Malaysia. Praeger, London

Loudon J 1966 Private stress and public ritual. Journal of Psychosomatics 10: 101–8

MacCormack C 1982 Health, fertility and birth in Moyamba District, Sierra Leone. In MacCormack C (ed.) Ethnography of fertility and birth. Academic Press, London, Ch 4

McGilvray D 1982 Sexual powers and fertility in Sri Lanka: Batticaloa Tamils and Moors. In MacCormack (ed.) Ethnography of fertility and birth. Academic Press, London, Ch 2

Oakley A 1979 Becoming a mother. Martin Robertson, Oxford

Oakley A 1980 Women confined. Towards a sociology of childbirth. Martin Robertson, Oxford

Okeley J 1977 Gypsy women: models in conflict. In Ardener S (ed.) Perceiving women. Halstead, New York, Ch 7

Palmer G 1988 The politics of breastfeeding. Pandora Press, London

Pillsbury B 1978 Doing the month: confinement and convalescence of Chinese women after childbirth. Social Science and Medicine 12: 11–112

Price A, Bamford N 1984 The breastfeeding guide for the working woman. Century, London

Reid M 1990 Pre-natal diagnosis and screening: a review. In Garcia J, Kilpatrick R, Richards M (eds) The politics of maternity care. Services for childbearing women in twentieth-century Britain. Clarendon Press, Oxford, Ch 16

Rothman B 1984 The meaning of choice in reproductive technology. In Arditti R, Klein R, Minden S (eds) Test-tube women: what future for motherhood? Pandora Press, London

Scheper-Hughes N 1991 Social indifference to child death. Lancet 337: 1144–6

Scheper-Hughes N 1992 Death without weeping. The violence of everyday life in Brazil. University of California Press, California

Steiner J 1989 How to survive as a working mother. Kogan Page, London

Stern G, Kruckman J 1983 Multi-disciplinary perspectives on post-partum depression: an anthropological critique. Social Science and Medicine 17(15): 1027–41

Thomson A 1989 Why don't women breastfeed? In Robinson S, Thomson A (eds) Midwives, research and childbirth. Chapman & Hall, London, Ch 11

Turner B 1990 Medical power and social knowledge. Sage, London

Turner V 1974 Dramas, fields and metaphors: symbolic action in human society. Cornell University Press, London

Turner V 1982 From ritual to theatre: The human seriousness of play. Performing Arts Journal, New York

United Kingdom Central Council for Nursing, Midwifery and Health Visiting 1993 Midwives rules. UKCC, London

Van Gennep A 1960 The rites of passage. Routledge & Kegan Paul, London

■ Suggested further reading

Browner C, Sargent C 1990 Anthropology and studies of human reproduction. In Thomas M, Sargent C (eds) Medical anthropology: contemporary theory and method. Praeger, London, Ch 12

Douglas M 1991 Purity and danger: an analysis of the concepts of pollution and taboo. Routledge, London

Freire P 1970 Pedagogy of the oppressed. Seabury, New York

MacCormack C 1982 Ethnography of Fertility and Birth. Academic Press, London

■ Useful addresses

La Lèche League of Great Britain
27 Old Gloucester Street
London WC1 6XX

National Childbirth Trust
9 Queensborough Terrace
London W2 3TB

The Working Mothers Association
77 Holloway Road
London N7 8JZ

Chapter 3

Injectable methods of pain relief in labour

Chris Bewley and Cliff Roberts

This chapter considers the use of pharmacological substances, principally opioids, given by injection for the relief of pain in labour where there are no complications, or when anaesthesia for operative or instrumental delivery is not required. The term 'injectable' is used to cover intramuscular, intravenous, epidural and intrathecal routes. The pharmacological action and physiological response of some drugs and their routes are explained, and current research evidence on maternal satisfaction, the effects on labour and side-effects in the mother and fetus/neonate over the short and long term is reviewed. Finally, suggestions are made for midwifery practice.

■ It is assumed that you are already aware of the following:

- The physiology of the first and second stages of labour;

- The physiology of pain transmission;

- Cultural, psychological and social factors affecting the perception of pain;

- The difference between analgesia and anaesthesia;

- UKCC guidance on drugs that can be administered by midwives.

■ Pain relief in labour

Beinart (1990) observes that, although the pain of childbirth is universally feared by women, it has only been during the 20th century that the use of drugs to relieve pain in labour has been seriously considered. She describes the search for appropriate drugs and routes of administration, documenting the rise and fall from favour of a number of substances and methods as their effects on mother and fetus became known. As this chapter will show, research into the effectiveness, safety and morbidity of currently available analgesia suggests that most methods have drawbacks for mother, fetus or both. Indeed, the World Health Organization is opposed to women receiving analgesia or anaesthesia in labour unless it is required to correct or prevent a complication in delivery (Wagner 1993).

☐ Midwives' attitudes to pain in labour

Niven (1994) found that, using a pain scale, midwives consistently scored women's pain lower than did the women themselves, even though when the woman scored herself highly, so did the midwife. Niven further suggests that underestimating women's pain is a protective mechanism to alleviate the distress that midwives may feel in the face of intractable pain. She also contends that midwives who have been nurses are used to administering potent and effective analgesics and are unprepared for the emotional trauma of being with a labouring woman whose pain is often not totally relieved. A study of Swedish midwives' attitudes to pain relief revealed a paradox, in that midwives felt that pharmacological methods of pain relief were overused, yet they continued to use them more frequently than non-pharmacological methods (Waldenstrom 1988).

The beneficial effects of a supportive birth companion are well documented, and Hodnett (1994) found that the need for pain relief was less if the woman was continuously supported by a trained person, even if she had not met that person before.

☐ The nature of labour pain

There is incomplete understanding of the causes of pain in labour (Dickersin 1989); most women experience pain, which may occur in the back, lower abdomen, thighs or suprapubic region. In the first stage of labour, pain results from myometrial contractions, which cause ischaemia in the uterus, and from dilatation of the cervix. When cervical dilatation is complete, pain results from stretching of the birth canal and, later, from pressure on the perineum (Heywood & Ho 1990). Labour pain is cyclical in nature, with peaks and troughs. The next section considers how knowledge of the physiology of pain in labour may influence the choice of analgesia.

☐ The physiology of pain in labour

Any sensation that produces pain is called a noxious stimulus, and the perception of such a noxious stimulus is termed nociception. Specific nerve endings (nociceptors) in the skin, subcutaneous tissues and viscera are sensitive to noxious stimuli and transmit impulses from the site of stimulation to the brain, where it is interpreted as pain. Nociceptors may be activated in two ways, chemically or mechanically. Substances known as chemical mediators occur naturally in the body; these include bradykinin (Ottoson 1983), prostaglandins, potassium, histamine and metabolic products, such as lactic acid, all of which activate the nociceptors and produce pain. Mechanical stimuli include overstretching, tearing, cutting and crushing. Sensations are transmitted by what is thought to be a nociceptive pathway.

	Fibre	Function
First order	A	Mechanoreceptor
	A delta and C	Nociceptor
		Mechanoreceptor
		Thermoreceptor
	Spinal column	**Function**
Second order	Spinothalamic tract	Nociception and temperature
	Dorsal column medial lemniscal	Touch and pressure
	Tract	**Function**
Third order	Thalamo-somatosensory cortex and widespread areas of the brain	Location of nociception

Figure 3.1 Neurons and their functions

■ Pain pathways

□ Ascending pathways

The primary or first order neurons (Figure 3.1) include the large-diameter primary afferents A alpha, beta and lambda and small-diameter primary afferents A delta and C fibres. Important structural features are diameter and myelination. The larger the diameter and thicker the myelination, the faster the transmission of impulses. Large, A delta fibres are thought to be responsible for acute, sharp pain, while unmyelinated C fibres give rise to dull, aching pain. All these fibres enter the dorsal horn and either synapse there or pass up the spinal column to the brain. The small-diameter primary afferents release substance P, a neurotransmitter thought to be responsible for the transmission of pain (Hinchliff & Montague 1988).

Second order neurons are those which ascend in the spinal pathways, the spinothalamic tract and the dorsal column medial lemniscal pathway.

Both pathways synapse and pass through the thalamus. There is also communication via the reticular activating system with the hypothalamus. The hypothalamus is responsible for governing the psychophysiological response to noxious stimuli in association with the cerebral cortex. The hypothalamus as part of the limbic system also modulates the emotional response. It also has under its control the autonomic nervous system, the neuroendocrine system and the endocrine system. It is therefore a central modulator of the psychological and physiological response to nociception.

Third order neurons arise from the thalamus and ultimately synapse within the cerebral cortex.

☐ Descending pathways

The crucial factor about descending pathways is that they are responsible for modulating the perception of noxious stimuli (Lewis & Liebeskind 1983). Enkephalin and serotonin are the major neurotransmitters in this pathway, and the main descending pathway is rich in endogenous opiate receptors. Activation of this pathway results in the release of enkephalin in the dorsal horn, which, via enkephalin receptors located on the small-diameter primary afferents, hyperpolarises the neurons and causes a reduction in the release of substance P, thereby reducing painful sensations.

☐ Gate control theory

Impulses are transmitted from the peripheral afferent fibres to the thalamus via transmission neurons arising in the dorsal horn. Neurons in the substantia gelatinosa of the dorsal horn act to inhibit or facilitate the transmission pathway. As well as transmitting painful stimuli, this pathway transmits input from touch receptors. The gate control theory (Melzack & Wall 1982) proposes that by activating touch receptors, which use large, A delta fibres, simultaneous transmission of painful stimuli by thin, C fibres will be blocked. The descending pathway and non-nociceptive afferents activate the inhibitory interneurons. This results in an effective increase in activity in the transmission neurons (Melzack & Wall 1982).

■ Neurophysiology of endorphins/receptors and the pharmacology of opioids

Opium, obtained from the opium poppy, has been used throughout the centuries for a number of reasons, including pain relief. It acts on the brain and spinal cord, reducing the perception of pain, and has the capacity to induce euphoria, analgesia and sleep. It contains papaverine, which is a smooth muscle relaxant. Opium derivatives include morphine and drugs closely related in structure to morphine, such as heroin and codeine. The term 'opioid' is used to describe any substance that produces morphine-like effects.

An understanding of the neuropharmacology of opioids and their receptors will enable the midwife to interpret the mode of action and the effects of any opioid substance used in practice.

☐ Agonists, antagonists and ligands

A ligand is any compound/drug, exogenous or endogenous, which binds to a specific receptor. This is referred to as ligand–receptor binding. A ligand that binds to its specific receptor and brings about a full physiological response is referred to as an agonist. A ligand that brings about a reduced or limited effect is termed a partial agonist. A ligand that abolishes the normal physiological response is referred to as an antagonist, that is, it will prevent a physiological response even in the presence of an agonist.

In the mid 1970s, substances were found within the body with varying opioid activity (Hughes *et al* 1975). These endogenous substances, termed opioids, have agonist activity at opioid receptors in various tissues in the nervous system, as described above. Opioids used by midwives and other health care professionals have their pharmacological activity on endogenous opioid receptors. Opioid derivatives include morphine itself, diamorphine, heroin and codeine. Synthetic derivatives include pethidine, fentanyl, pentazocine, cyclazocine and others. Nalorphine and levallorphan are partial agonists at opioid receptors, while naloxone is a full antagonist. Thus these agents can be used when necessary to reverse the effects of opioids in cases of maternal or fetal side-effects or overdose.

The cellular effects of opioids are not well understood but are thought to include antagonism of adenylate cyclase activity and an increase in potassium conductance. The resulting hyperpolarisation reduces the influx of calcium via electrically gated channels at the nerve terminals, with the result that less substance P is released.

Opioid receptors are classified as mu, delta, kappa, sigma and epsilon. These classifications are important in pharmacology as efforts are made to produce drugs that can activate specific receptors for pain relief without activating those which produce side-effects. Three receptors produce the main pharmacological effects.

☐ Mu receptors

Agonists include opioids, beta-endorphin and enkephalin. The mu receptors facilitate supraspinal analgesia but are associated with respiratory depression, euphoria and physical dependence (Trounce 1994). Naloxone is an antagonist.

☐ Kappa receptors

Kappa receptor agonists include dynorphin. These receptors facilitate spinal analgesia and are associated with pupillary constriction and sedation. Norbinaltorphimine is a selective antagonist.

☐ Sigma receptors

The sigma receptor may not be a legitimate opiate receptor as non-opioid substances such as haloperidol have agonist activity and agonists are not reversed by naloxone. Activation of these receptors by opioids is thought to cause dysphoria and hallucinations.

☐ Morphine

Morphine has been identified as a major pain-relieving drug; it is metabolised in the liver via conjugation with glucuronide and excreted in bile and urine as morphine glucuronide. Morphine crosses the placenta, and, as neonates have a low conjugating capacity as a result of their immature livers, the unwanted effects of morphine, including the depression of consciousness, respiratory function and cardiovascular function, persist for much longer than in an adult. Morphine is not, therefore, the opiate of choice in labour.

The addictive nature of morphine and its analogues has led to a search for a non-addictive synthetic derivative, which has resulted in the production of pethidine, fentanyl, methadone, pentazocine and cyclazocine, although these drugs may also induce dependency.

☐ Pethidine

Pethidine has one tenth the potency of morphine, with a virtually identical pharmacological action. Its duration of action is much shorter than that of morphine. Following intramuscular injection, the onset of action is around 15 minutes and is maximal in 1.0–1.5 hours. It can be given every 2–3 hours. Naloxone will reverse about 80 per cent of the respiratory depressant effects of pethidine. Metabolism is via N-demethylation in the liver rather than glucuronidation. The fetal liver is able to cope with this method of elimination, and any drug passed through the placenta is quickly metabolised. Hallucinogenic and convulsant effects are seen owing to the production in the liver of norpethidine. Drug interactions have occurred with monoamine oxidase inhibitors, resulting in maternal hyperthermia, hyperexcitability and convulsions (Trounce 1994).

Pethidine has long been used for pain relief in labour and is available for use in hospital and community settings for midwives to give intramuscularly, usually on a standing order. Its maternal side-effects have been well documented and include nausea and vomiting, delayed gastric emptying, respiratory depression, depression of the central nervous system, drowsiness and postural hypotension. For the woman, respiratory depression lowers blood oxygen levels and increases carbon dioxide levels, which may not be recovered between contractions, adversely affecting fetal oxygenation. She may also be less able to take an active physical or psychological role in labour and therefore be denied a satisfactory role in the birth experience. Thomson and Hillier (1994) reviewed literature on the influence of pethidine on the length of first and second stages of labour, their paper suggesting that pethidine increases the length of both of these stages. However, they point out that, owing to methodological flaws and small sample sizes, the research did not categorically confirm this.

Adverse effects on the fetus and neonate are also well documented, particularly when delivery occurs within 2–3 hours of the woman having received pethidine, thus exposing the fetus to the maximum effect during delivery itself (Savona-Ventura *et al* 1991). Pethidine is implicated in a loss of variability of fetal heart rate, neonatal asphyxia and a delay in breastfeeding due to drowsiness (Rajan 1994; Nissen *et al* 1995). It has also been postulated that it may predispose to drug addiction in later life due to 'imprinting' (Jacobson *et al* 1990).

In terms of maternal satisfaction, MacArthur *et al*'s (1993) retrospective study of 11 701 women suggested that 20.7 per cent of those who used pethidine were 'fully satisfied' with it, although 3.5 per cent of those who were 'fully satisfied' felt that pethidine had deprived them of the pleasure of giving birth. Priest and Rosser (1991) suggest that, although some women derive pain relief from pethidine, many women dislike the associated feelings of detachment and loss of control.

Patient-controlled administration (PCA) of pethidine is possible via the intravenous route; Rayburn *et al* (1989) compared two groups of labouring women, one using PCA and the other receiving 3-hourly intravenous pethidine as a bolus dose from a nurse. Overall, maternally administered total dosages were higher, yet pain relief was judged to be similar in both groups. The researchers concluded that the higher dosages in self-administration may pose an increased risk to the fetus.

☐ Fentanyl

Fentanyl is a derivative of pethidine and is much more potent. It is very short acting and its effects are similar to those of pethidine. It is also a potent respiratory depressant (Trounce 1994). Recently, it has been used in conjunction with local anaesthetics in epidural analgesia (Thorp & Breedlove 1996) and spinal analgesia, since fentanyl does not affect motor neuron activity. The combination uses lower doses of local anaesthetic to produce analgesia of rapid onset and longer duration than can be achieved using local anaesthetic alone, yet there is no ensuing weakness in the lower limbs (Fernando 1995).

☐ Heroin

Heroin (diamorphine hydrochloride) is used during labour in Scotland and in some parts of Northern England (Robinson 1995). Heroin is an ester of morphine; it has a short half-life, and, as well as having powerful pain-relieving properties, it produces feelings of euphoria. Side-effects are depression of the cough reflex and of the respiratory centre in mother and fetus. There are suggestions that use during labour may predispose to addiction of the child in later life (Jacobson *et al* 1990).

☐ Meptid (meptazinol)

Whereas morphine and pethidine are full agonists, meptazinol is a partial agonist, which acts as a powerful analgesic but is less likely to cause euphoria or respiratory depression (Trounce 1994). Sheikh and Tunstall (1986) conclude that, when used during labour, there is little difference between meptazinol and pethidine in terms of pain relief and side-effects in mother and baby. However, its duration of action is shorter, and women generally experienced greater feelings of nausea.

■ Methods of administration, advantages and disadvantages

The opioids are highly lipid soluble and are well distributed throughout the body water compartments. This means that the drug is capable of breaching the blood–brain and placental barriers. Ideally, a drug used for pain relief in labour should not cross the placenta because of potential adverse effects on the fetus. In terms of the mother, while the aim is to block the transmission of nociception in the dorsal horn by inhibiting small primary afferents, large primary afferents and central neurons in the brain can be adversely affected by circulating opioids. Logically, the most appropriate approach would be to expose only the small primary afferents to the effects of opioids. In order to do this, opioids need to be highly localised in the dorsal horn area and at a dose sufficient to inhibit small-fibre but not larger fibre transmission. Clearly, the systemic route of administration by oral or intramuscular routes can never achieve this aim. However, the epidural route used under the right circumstances can.

☐ Epidural analgesia

The aim of spinal analgesia is to block pain transmitted by small primary afferents while not affecting sensation and motor activity, which is transmitted by larger fibres.

Drugs given via the epidural route are deposited extradurally, that is, they are deposited in the extradural space (see below). From here, they will diffuse into the cerebrospinal fluid (CSF).

Impulses from nerve fibres are blocked in the following order:

1. Autonomic preganglionic B fibres;

2. Cold, then warm, temperature fibres;

3. Pinprick fibres;

4. Fibres conveying pain greater than pinprick;

5. Touch fibres;

6. Deep pressure fibres;

7. Somatic motor fibres;

8. Fibres conveying vibration and proprioreception (movement).

Epidural infusion allows the diffusion of drugs (opioids, local anaesthetics or a combination of the two) to the posterior sensory root ganglia. In the absence of any of the complications or side-effects, discussed below, epidural analgesia produces a minimum of systemic effects. Some drugs will, however, enter the CSF, diffuse into the surrounding tissues or enter the venous drainage system. Advantages of the epidural route include effective analgesia with the minimum of other sensory and motor disruption (Fernando 1995).

Disadvantages include variable control of pain when bolus top-ups are used, the risk of catheter migration into the epidural vein or subarachnoid space, and side-effects such as urinary retention, sedation, nausea, itching and hypotension. Epidural analgesia also requires skilled, experienced anaesthetists and midwives to set up and maintain the infusion, and to observe both mother and fetus for signs of side-effects. Mander (1993) suggests that the advent of epidural analgesia created the need for a whole new group of professionals in the form of obstetric anaesthetists.

In the 1970s epidural analgesia was hailed as a revolutionary method of pain relief that would enable all women to have a painless labour and delivery (Beinart 1990). There was intensive campaigning to ensure that all women would have access to epidural analgesia, especially as some maternity units were only able to offer the service during the day, when appropriately experienced anaesthetists were on duty (Mander 1993). Kitzinger's (1987) international survey of National Childbirth Trust members was one of the first to suggest that epidural analgesia might be a source of maternal dissatis-faction with labour and might also be implicated in physical sequelae, including headache, backache and urinary problems. Her findings, although deemed methodologically flawed because the sample was self-selected and unrandomised, were supported by other work (MacArthur *et al* 1990, 1992; MacLeod *et al* 1995; Benhamou *et al* 1995). MacArthur *et al's* (1990) findings of post-delivery nerve and musculoskeletal problems further suggested that an epidural, by blocking the sensations of positional discom-fort that would otherwise have caused women to change position, led them to maintain positions giving rise to damage. Mander (1994) reviews studies of epidural use, noting that epidural anaesthesia leads to longer labours and higher rates of intervention and suggesting that relaxation of the pelvic floor prevents rotation of the fetal head, especially in the second stage.

Morgan and Kadim (1994) sought a method of epidural anaesthesia that would eliminate pain but not sensation, so that women would be able to mobilise and respond to physical sensations in labour, yet remain pain free. Morgan pioneered the so-called walking or mobile epidural and claimed a lower caesarean section rate using this method than conventional methods. Morgan and Kadim (1994) also suggest that the use of smaller size spinal needles and more experienced anaesthetists has reduced the incidence of dural puncture and other previously recorded adverse effects of epidurals.

The use and effects of epidural analgesia demand ongoing research. Thorp and Breedlove's (1996) evaluation of studies and articles on epidural anaesthesia from 1970 to 1995 concludes that, although it is an effective method of pain relief in labour, it is associated with maternal fever, increased intervention for fetal distress and longer labours. They are cautious about linking epidural with chronic backache, as is Reynolds (1995), who contends that a number of adverse postnatal complications, including backache and footdrop, are wrongly attributed to epidural analgesia and that these conditions can arise from intrapelvic neuropathy resulting from lumbar or sacral nerve damage, which may occur even in a spontaneous delivery without epidural anaesthesia.

As far as midwives are concerned, much of the debate surrounding epidural anaesthesia relates to medical and anaesthetic practices. However, to provide appropriate information for women to make informed choices, midwives must be familiar with the debates surrounding techniques and side-effects. Informed consent depends on the woman having the appropriate information on which to base her decision. A postal question-naire survey by Bush (1995) led to the view that the information on which women based their informed consent for obstetric anaesthesia and analgesia could be improved.

In midwifery practice, midwives must be aware of local policies on epidurals, including the drugs used and the midwifery action to be taken in the event of side-effects or complications. Midwives must also know the dosage and routes of administration of drugs used to reverse the side-effects, and they must be competent in maternal and neonatal resuscitation.

■ Conclusion

None of the methods of injectable pain relief reviewed is consistently capable of eliminating pain without some other physical or psychological effect on the mother or fetus. Midwives' time is taken up in the administration of drugs and the technology surrounding epidural anaesthesia, when evidence suggests that midwives' continued physical presence with a labouring woman reduces the need for pharmacological pain relief. Nevertheless, many women still look for pain relief in labour, and more research is needed to find a safe, acceptable method of pain relief, be it pharmacological or non-pharmacological, to help women to cope with labour pain.

■ Recommendations for clinical practice in the light of currently available evidence

1. Midwives need to come to terms with their own feelings when confronted with a woman in pain, so that they do not use drugs to ease their own feelings of helplessness.

2. More research is needed to find a safe method of pain relief in labour for those women who want it.

3. Babies of mothers who wish to breastfeed and who have received pethidine should spend longer in close contact with mothers until they establish a rooting reflex.

4. Midwives should use naloxone to reverse the effects of opioids where appropriate.

■ Practice check

● How much pethidine do you give in one dose to labouring women? When do you give it? Have you thought of lowering the dose?

● Do you have ready access to an up to date copy of the *British National Formulary*?

● How often are you able to give one-to-one support to women in labour?

● Do you find that attending to the technology involved in epidural analgesia takes precedence over the development of a supportive relationship with a labouring woman?

● Are you familiar with the drugs currently used for epidural analgesia and their side-effects?

■ References

Beinart J 1990 Obstetric analgesia and the control of childbirth. In Garcia J, Kilpatrick R, Richards M (eds) The politics of maternity care. Clarendon, Oxford, Ch 6

Benhamou D, Hamza J, Ducot B 1995 Post-partum headache after epidural analgesia without dural puncture. International Journal of Obstetric Anaesthesia 4: 44–7

Bush D 1995 A comparison of informed consent for obstetric anaesthesia in the USA and UK. International Journal of Obstetric Anaesthesia 4: 1–6

Dickersin K 1989 Pharmacological control of pain during labour. In Chalmers I Enkin M, Keirse MJNC (eds) Effective care in pregnancy and childbirth. Oxford University Press, Oxford, Ch 57

Fernando R 1995 Mobile epidurals for labour analgesia. Maternal and Child Health 20(11): 353–8

Heywood AM, Ho E 1990 Pain relief in labour. In Alexander J, Levy V, Roch S (eds) Intrapartum care: a research-based approach. Macmillan, London, Ch 5

Hinchliff S, Montague V 1988 Physiology for nursing practice. Baillière Tindall, London

Hodnett ED 1994 Support from caregivers during childbirth. In Enkin MW, Keirse MJNC, Renfrew MJ, Neilson JP (eds) Pregnancy and childbirth. Cochrane Database of Systematic Reviews no. 03871, Oxford

Hughes J, Smith T, Morgan B, Fothergill L 1975 Purification and properties of enkephalin – the possible endogenous ligand for the morphine receptor. Life Sciences 16: 1753–8

Jacobson B, Nyberg K, Grondbladh L 1990 Opiate addiction in adult offspring through possible imprinting after obstetric treatment. British Medical Journal 301(6760): 1067–70

Kitzinger S 1987 Some women's experiences of epidurals – a descriptive study. National Childbirth Trust, London

Lewis J, Liebeskind J 1983 Pain suppressive systems of the brain. Trends in Pharmacological Sciences 4: 73–5

MacArthur C, Lewis M, Knox EG 1992 Investigation of long term problems after obstetric epidural anaesthesia. British Medical Journal 304: 1279–82

MacArthur C, Lewis M, Knox EG 1993 Evaluation of obstetric analgesia and anaesthesia: long term maternal recollections. International Journal of Obstetric Anesthesia 2(1): 3–11

MacArthur C, Lewis M, Knox EG, Crawford JS 1990 Epidural anaesthesia and long term backache after childbirth. British Medical Journal 301: 9–11

MacLeod J, Macintyre C, McClure JH, Whitefield A 1995 Backache and epidural anaesthesia. International Journal of Obstetric Anaesthesia 4: 21–5

Mander R 1993 Epidural analgesia, 1, Recent history. British Journal of Midwifery 6: 259–63

Mander R 1994 Epidural analgesia, 2, Research basis. British Journal of Midwifery 2(1): 12–16

Melzack R, Wall P 1982 The challenge of pain. Penguin, London

Morgan BM, Kadim MY 1994 Mobile regional analgesia. British Journal of Obstetrics and Gynaecology 101(10): 839–41

Nissen E, Lilja G, Mattiesen AS 1995 Effects of maternal pethidine on infants' developing breast feeding behaviour. Acta Paediatrica 84(2): 140–5

Niven C 1994 Coping with labour pain: the midwife's role. In Robinson S, Thomson A (eds) Midwives research and childbirth, vol. 3. Chapman & Hall, London, Ch 5

Ottoson D 1983 Physiology of the nervous system. Oxford University Press, New York

Priest J, Rosser J 1991 Pethidine – a shot in the dark. MIDIRS Midwifery Digest 4: 373–5 (editorial)

Rajan L 1994 The impact of obstetric procedures and analgesia/anaesthesia during labour and delivery on breast feeding. Midwifery 10(2): 87–103

Rayburn W, Leuschen MP, Earl R 1989 Intravenous meperedine during labour: a randomised comparison between nursing and patient controlled administration. Obstetrics and Gynecology 74(5): 702–6

Reynolds F 1995 Maternal sequelae of childbirth. British Journal of Anaesthesia 75(5): 515–17

Robinson J 1995 Use of heroin in labour – AIMS concern. AIMS Journal 7(2): 9–10

Savona-Ventura C, Sammut M, Sammut C 1991 Pethidine blood concentrations at time of birth. International Journal of Obstetrics and Gynecology 36(2): 103–7

Sheikh A, Tunstall ME 1986 Comparative study of meptazinol and pethidine for the relief of pain in labour. British Journal of Obstetrics and Gynaecology 93(3): 264–9

Thomson AM, Hillier VF 1994 A re-evaluation of the effect of pethidine on the length of labour. Journal of Advanced Nursing 19(3): 448–56

Thorp JA, Breedlove G 1996 Epidural analgesia in labor: an evaluation of risks and benefits. Birth 23(2): 63–83

Trounce J 1994 Clinical pharmacology for nurses. Churchill Livingstone, London

Wagner M 1993 Research shows medication of pain is not safe. Caduceus 20: 14–15; reprinted in MIDIRS Midwifery Digest 4: 307–9

Waldenstrom U 1988 Midwives' attitudes to pain relief during labour and delivery. Midwifery 4(2): 48–57

Chapter 4

Active management of labour

Sue McDonald

The birth experience and the events that surround it have become a major source of discussion, debate and evaluation over the past decade. This has addressed not only the physical process of giving birth, but also the psychological impact of birth on women. There is now a growing demand among parents for information about available options and participation in decisions related to place of birth, choice of carer and models of care as well as the level of intervention during pregnancy and labour. The information desired may cover ultrasound screening, elective caesarean section, the induction of labour and the attachment of fetal monitoring aids, or whether the administration of an oxytocic for management of the third stage of labour is necessary. Expertise in interpreting current trends and research evidence is vital for clinicians and, in turn, requires time to obtain and review the ever-increasing amount of information prior to its dissemination in an appropriate form to women and their supporters. The aim of this chapter is to explore the concept of active management of labour, its origins and its application to current labour care.

■ It is assumed that you are already aware of the following:

● The process and definition of 'normal labour';

● The policies of your unit relating to when to intervene in labour.

■ Background

At the turn of the century, poor nutrition resulting in rickets was a major contributor to a high incidence of pelvic contracture among women of childbearing age. With the virtual disappearance of pelvic contracture in economically developed countries midway through the 20th century, there was an expectation that the caesarean section rate would also decline (Olah & Neilson 1994). This, however, does not seem to have been the case.

In the mid 1960s O'Driscoll and colleagues introduced a multifaceted approach to the management of labour (referred to as active management) in nulliparous women at the National Maternity Hospital, Dublin, in the belief that 'Prolonged labour presented a picture of mental anguish and physical morbidity which often leads to a surgical intervention and may produce a permanent revulsion to childbirth' (O'Driscoll *et al* 1969).

This management strategy focused on women having their first birth as 'The fundamental differences between a first birth are so great that primigravidae and multigravidae behave as different biological species'. Indeed, 'A woman's first birth experience is of paramount importance as it determines the attitude to all subsequent births'. Furthermore, 'A first labour is unique and the sequence of events that takes place on that occasion has no relevance to later births. The lesson is simple: provide a high level of care and attention the first time round and women will require little attention on the next occasion. Conversely, the damage inflicted by a low level of care and attention first time round is usually irreversible' (O'Driscoll & Meagher 1986).

The components of active management as prescribed in the Dublin management protocol were:

- Antenatal preparation/education;

- Early amniotomy;

- Correction of an abnormal labour pattern with oxytocin in the first and second stages of labour;

- Continuous support during labour.

Adherence to this protocol was designed to ensure that no woman would be undelivered by the end of 24 hours. This time frame in more recent years has been modified to reflect an expectation that the majority of women would be delivered within 12 hours of the onset of labour (O'Driscoll 1993). The Dublin regime stresses the importance of an accurate diagnosis of labour prior to early amniotomy and/or the implementation of other facets of an active management policy in order to avoid other complications, such as the misdiagnosis of prolonged labour, which may in turn lead to interventions such as instrumental birth or a caesarean section. The caesarean section rate in Dublin at the time of introducing this management policy in 1969 was approximately 4 per cent (O'Driscoll *et al* 1969) and, according to Lopez-Zeno *et al* (1992), has altered little since.

In the past two decades, medical technology has advanced at an unprecedented pace, with the introduction of and an increased frequency in the use of (even a reliance upon) pregnancy and labour assessment tools such as ultrasound and fetal heart rate monitoring, which are designed for the detection of abnormal occurrences. Intertwined with this has been an improvement in neonatal surveillance technology and clinical expertise. This progress has meant that babies of much lower gestational age are being given an increased chance of survival and women with medical complications of pregnancy such as diabetes and hypertension a more favourable pregnancy outcome. It was also anticipated that, by appropriate screening for early detection of problems, the increased use of surveillance equipment would be justified by a reduction in the number of caesarean section births. However, in spite of, or perhaps owing to, this increased use of technology, the caesarean section rate has steadily increased, figures in excess of 20 per cent of total births in parts of the USA and Australia being quoted (Turnbull & Laing 1995).

Shearer (1989), commenting on the rate of caesarean section reaching 25 per cent in the USA, expressed the importance of clinicians acknowledging that this was not a result of a higher number of sicker mothers and babies. Rather, it was due to the view that birth was a medical problem to be managed medically and that, as long as this view remained unchallenged, the problem of unnecessary interventions would not change. Shearer issued a challenge to obstetric training programmes to teach about normal labour first, along with the importance of how and why to communicate with parents, the value of true informed consent as a process, and the teaching of an attitude of healthy scepticism towards the limits of technology (Shearer 1989).

In 1989 Boylan described active management as being the active involvement of the consultant obstetrician in decisions made about the course of labour for all women entering the delivery ward regardless of the risk status of their pregnancy. This has remained the consistent philosophy behind the policy of care developed and implemented in Ireland and described by O'Driscoll *et al* (1969), and is the basis on which current policies are made in maternity units around the world where active management is practised.

Since the 1960s many aspects of labour care have been studied. However, several of the components of the active management policy described above (for example, amniotomy and the oxytocic augmentation of labour) have been readily incorporated into obstetric practice all over the world since the late 1970s, despite the fact that this policy of care had not been subjected to any scientific evaluation. Perhaps, as in many other areas of pregnancy and labour care, individual components of care or procedures that have in themselves been shown to be effective have been meshed together in clinical practice until there exists a 'package' of care that has been gradually adopted into routine practice.

Opponents of active management have disputed claims that this type of management is responsible for a reduction in the rate of instrumental delivery and argue that amniotomy increases the infection risk, that even in first labours oxytocin occasionally causes fetal hypoxia and maternal hyponatraemia, and that many women resent the interventions (Thornton & Lilford 1994). Certainly, during the 1980s, Inch (1985) challenged the necessity for some procedures such as artificial rupture of the membranes, the use of oxytocics to induce or augment labour, the use of fetal monitors and the administration of oxytocics in the third stage (in essence, active management), which appeared to have become routinely associated with labour. The mechanisms and interrelationships of all these procedures can be poorly understood in some cases by both the pregnant women and by the clinicians providing their care.

Although the perinatal mortality rate has fallen with no obvious increase in infection, there has been a steady rise in the number of caesarean sections and instrumental deliveries.

■ Antenatal preparation/education

Part of the philosophy of the original 'package' of active management was to 'define a woman's role in labour and to teach her how to fulfil it' (O'Driscoll *et al* 1969). This it seems was to be achieved by '*teaching* her by giving a broad understanding of the birth process and *training* her how to achieve the ultimate prize of a spontaneous delivery' (O'Driscoll *et al* 1969). It may be generally accepted that the education process must involve the consumers to whom the care is being offered (or, in some cases on whom it is being imposed). However, I believe that many women would find the Dublin antenatal education method unusual. O'Driscoll *et al* (1969) describe the process used to assist women to feel less anxious about labour. Their understanding of what can be expected on arrival at the hospital in labour is tested in a direct question and answer format:

> QUESTION: How will you know when to go to hospital?
> ANSWER: When I get painful contractions which resemble period pains, together with a show or persistent leakage of water – or, failing either of these, when the pains come at regular intervals of 10 minutes or less.
> QUESTION: How long will you be there before the baby is born?
> ANSWER: Six hours on average, never longer than 12.
> QUESTION: Will you ever be left alone?
> ANSWER: Never.
>
> (O'Driscoll *et al* 1969)

The dialogue and attitude used by clinicians in the provision of information can be as powerful as the written text. It has the potential for a significant impact on influencing the way in which women interpret information and make decisions about their individual preferences for pregnancy and childbirth. The Dublin approach to discussion is one way to achieve the desired outcome. Some may prefer a more individual approach, such as the recently released Informed Choice Leaflets produced in the UK by MIDIRS and the NHS Centre for Reviews and Dissemination (MIDIRS/NHS 1996). There are leaflets for health professionals and separate leaflets on the same topic written in plain language for consumers. Each leaflet contains evidence-based information about the benefits or limited use of some aspects of pregnancy and childbirth care for women and health professionals. The acceptability and practical application of these leaflets in the community setting is currently being evaluated.

While the leaflets are a major step forward in providing women, their partners and clinicians with well-balanced information, they should not be seen as a substitute for personal communication. They are likely to be of limited value if not offered in the context of continuing interactive support and co-operation between the women and the professionals providing pregnancy and childbirth care. It is important that, in situations in which the leaflets are used, the organisation makes a commitment to ensuring that the options discussed within them are available and accessible to all women.

■ Identification of the onset of labour

The 1969 Dublin definition of 'diagnosis of labour' required there to be painful uterine contractions accompanied by a 'show', spontaneous rupture of the membranes or dilatation of the cervix (O'Driscoll *et al* 1969). By 1989 in the same hospital, the diagnosis was described as being based on painful contractions with or without a 'show', tremendous importance being placed on cervical dilatation in first labours as the nulliparous cervix effaces before it begins to dilate at the onset of labour (Boylan 1989). Yet there still seems to be a variation in what authors of different studies consider to be the most important elements for a definite diagnosis of labour, including regular painful contractions and some effacement and/or ruptured membranes, or contractions, effacement and dilatation.

How is the onset of labour correctly identified? Is it assumed that all women will present with the same history and go through labour in the same way and, more importantly, that all clinicians involved in the initial and subsequent physical assessment of an individual woman during the course of labour will interpret their clinical findings in the same way? DeMott and Sandmire (1992) emphasised the importance of awaiting the active phase of labour in order to avoid a misdiagnosis that may ultimately lead to increased levels of intervention such as caesarean section. This was in support of Porreco (1990), who stated that failure to progress was really failure to wait for the onset of active labour.

In the midst of all this confusion is the woman. If clinicians cannot agree on a definition for labour, what chance does the labouring (or perhaps not labouring!) woman have?

According to Bonovich (1990), between 10 and 20 per cent of women presenting to a 500-bed community hospital with signs of early labour were sent home undelivered. A randomised trial was undertaken comparing a group of women who were assigned to receive either exposure to an educational technique aimed at teaching women how to recognise the onset of labour, or the usual routine instructions about when to present to the labour ward. The results showed a significant decrease in the number of unnecessary visits made to the labour ward by women in the experimental group. Interpretation of the results should, however, be viewed with caution as the randomisation process produced an uneven distribution of age, educational level, age of the father of the fetus and household size. This resulted in the experimental group being older and better educated, having older partners and living in smaller households, all of which may influence the woman's ability to learn and cope with labour.

■ Early amniotomy

There are areas of practice in which finding a balance of care between meeting women's preferences for a more minimal intervention approach to childbirth and those of clinicians, who advocate a more active management approach, has presented some dilemmas.

The timing of when a woman feels the need to come into the hospital labour ward may influence the attending doctor's decision to induce or augment labour. Early presentation with perceived signs of the onset of labour or spontaneous rupture of the membranes in the absence of contractions may in some cases create the potential for an increase in the use of procedures such as external fetal monitoring, surgical rupture of membranes or the initiation of intravenous oxytocin.

The published literature reveals that few trials have been conducted on the efficacy of early amniotomy and that those which have been conducted have been small and of insecure methodological quality (Keirse 1995).

■ Oxytocin induction and augmentation

Keirse (1995) published an overview of three trials comparing a policy of starting intravenous oxytocin at the time when the membranes were artificially ruptured with its commencement after a few hours if labour had not commenced. Although the trials were of variable methodological quality, two of the trials showed that women who received oxytocin from the time of the amniotomy were statistically significantly more likely to have delivered within 12 hours and within 24 hours than those who had amniotomy alone, and less likely to be delivered by caesarean section or forceps. Furthermore, fewer women in the amniotomy and oxytocin group had operative deliveries in the presence of maternal pyrexia or offensive smelling liquor. Those infants whose mothers received the policy of amniotomy plus oxytocin at induction were less likely to have depressed Apgar scores, although this result was statistically significant in only one of the studies.

A variation on the above situation is that of the woman who presents at term with ruptured membranes but whose contractions have not commenced. Does waiting for the spontaneous onset of labour increase the risk of maternal and fetal infection? A large, multicentre, randomised controlled trial involving over 5000 women was undertaken by Hannah *et al* (1996). The purpose of the trial was to compare induction of labour with expectant management for prelabour rupture of the membranes at term. Women who had consented to take part in the trial and met prespecified inclusion criteria were randomly allocated to receive one of four management protocols:

- Induction with oxytocin;

- Induction with prostaglandins;

- Expectant management and then oxytocin induction/augmentation if required; *or*

- Expectant management and then prostaglandin induction/ augmentation if required.

The results of this study are of major importance. In summary, it was found that:

- The rates of neonatal infection were similar in all study groups;

- Caesarean section rates were similar across the groups;

- Chorioamnionitis was less likely to be found in the induction-with-oxytocin group;

- Maternal postpartum infection rates were lower in the induction-with-oxytocin group.

While it would appear that a woman could reasonably, on the basis of these results, weigh up the slightly increased risk of infection against what she might perceive as being a more unpleasant experience in the procedure of induction, it should be remembered that there were four stillbirth/ neonatal deaths in the expectant management group. While not statistically significant, this outcome is of serious consequence and should not be ignored or discounted when discussing the risks and benefits of a management policy with women who are seeking to make informed decisions about options in pregnancy and labour care.

There are two published trials in the literature that are prospective randomised controlled trials of active management compared with routine labour management (Frigoletto *et al* 1992; Lopez-Zeno *et al* 1992). In the first, Lopez-Zeno *et al* were concerned that the incidence of caesarean section was increasing as a result of an increased number of diagnoses of dystocia (arrest of labour). The aim of their study was therefore to test the programme of active management to ascertain whether applying the elements of accurate diagnosis of the onset of labour, early amniotomy and oxytocin infusion if necessary would increase the number of vaginal births. The study did not test the effect of continuous professional support during labour. Nulliparous women in spontaneous labour at term were randomly allocated to receive either active management or traditional management, that is, artificial rupture of membranes, the use of oxytocin and the provision of continuous support at the discretion of the attending clinicians. There was a 26 per cent reduction in the number of caesarean sections as a result of dystocia for women in the active management group. The authors acknowledged that, as the study was not blinded, this may have resulted in a 'drift in the management of labour towards a more active approach, thereby contributing to a lower caesarean section rate for this group as well' (Lopez-Zeno *et al* 1992).

The second study was undertaken in the USA. Frigoletto *et al* were also concerned by their hospital's escalating caesarean section rate of beyond 20 per cent. A totally separate labour ward was constructed, well distanced from the current labour ward, so little 'contamination' from staff interaction was encountered. Staff for this new ward were specially trained in the 'Dublin' active management protocol. The currently operating labour ward continued management in the usual way (that is, no constraints were placed on the management practices of physicians caring for women in labour). The results of the trial showed there to be no difference in the rate of the primary outcome of caesarean section between the two management protocols. The median duration of labour was 2.7 hours shorter and the rate of maternal fever lower in the active management group. The major factor that differed between the protocols of the two labour wards was the aspect of continuous professional support in labour. An important factor to be considered is perhaps that the Dublin regime, in recognising the importance of continuous midwifery support, captured the essential component of labour care that results in fewer operative births, and that applying active management policies that do not encompass continuous midwifery support are unlikely to attain the same success rate. It is unfortunate that a randomised controlled trial was not undertaken prior to the Dublin active management policy being implemented to evaluate how many of the women in the Dublin population would have delivered vaginally within the same time frame but without the rigid active management policy.

■ Continuous support in labour

The continuous presence of a midwife has long been considered to be a vital part of labour care. Although early amniotomy following the diagnosis of labour, the use of oxytocic agents to facilitate labour and the implementation of partograms to monitor the progress of labour have been readily adopted in labour ward practice, the majority of busy maternity units do not have one midwife to each labouring woman, particularly during the early phase of labour. This situation should perhaps be reviewed. A perceived benefit of continuous support may be in providing not only emotional support, but also the potential to facilitate a more active approach to birth by promoting ambulation and the simple practical measure of ensuring that an adequate fluid and nutritional intake is maintained. Attention to these factors in the early phase of labour may be the key to the alleviation of anxiety and the adjustment to the progress of labour, thereby reducing the need for operative delivery.

A range of pain management strategies, such as immersion in water, transcutaneous electrical nerve stimulation (TENS), inhalational analgesia, homoeopathic therapies, relaxation techniques and intramuscular analgesia, may be employed, with a resultant reduction in the use of epidural analgesia, which, while it has been shown to provide effective pain relief, is also more likely to be associated with an instrumental delivery (Howell 1995). See also Chapter 3 in this volume.

■ Third stage of labour

Debate about the active management of labour also extends to the third stage. This is discussed in more detail in Chapter 8 in this volume.

■ Continuous fetal monitoring

It would be difficult to complete this chapter without making some comment on the contribution of fetal monitoring to the concept of active management over the last decade or so.

Once intervention, such as oxytocin infusion, occurs, women are no longer considered to be at low risk. The attending medical practitioner frequently wishes to 'monitor' labour more closely and thus begins the well-described 'cascade of interventions' (Mold & Stein 1986). This can involve the application of continuous fetal monitoring, restricting the woman's freedom of movement, increasing the risk of a longer first stage of labour and increasing the likelihood of epidural analgesia, a longer second stage, operative vaginal delivery and caesarean section. Inch (1985) also applied the concept to third stage management of labour.

At least ten randomised controlled trials of continuous fetal monitoring versus intermittent auscultation have shown that continuous fetal monitoring results in higher instrumental delivery and caesarean section rates. The recently compiled series of Informed Choice Leaflets (published by MIDIRS and the NHS Centre for Reviews and Dissemination) reviews the evidence, citing two studies in particular (Haverkamp *et al* 1976; Kelso *et al* 1978) that claim an increased caesarean section rate of 160 per cent if continuous fetal monitoring alone is performed and an increase of 30 per cent if such monitoring is carried out in conjunction with fetal scalp blood sampling. There is no evidence that intensive fetal monitoring without fetal scalp blood sampling for pH reduces the risk of a low Apgar score or the need for admission to neonatal nurseries. The only neonatal outcome that appears to be improved is that of neonatal seizure when labour has been induced or augmented with oxytocin at term and a combination of continuous fetal monitoring and fetal scalp blood sampling has been used. The type of seizure experienced in these infants does not, however, appear to be associated with long-term impairment (Neilson 1995).

A study of women's views of continuous fetal monitoring versus intermittent auscultation conducted as part of the Dublin randomised controlled trial of intrapartum fetal heart rate monitoring suggested that 'the method of monitoring was less important to the women in the trial than the support and reassurance they received from staff and companions' (Garcia *et al* 1985). The results of this study indicated that women in the continuous monitoring arm of the study were more likely to be left alone for short periods. These results were consistent with the results of other randomised controlled trials and observational studies.

The question of what happens in units where this level of technology is not readily available or there are not the staff sufficiently skilled in interpreting the results of fetal monitoring traces has not as yet been answered. Further research is required to address this issue.

■ Summary

Active management is a policy of care that has been introduced into obstetric and subsequently midwifery practice without the benefit of scientific evaluation. While there is, without doubt, a place for more structured and formalised procedures for care of women who are at higher risk of complications, for example women with prolonged rupture of the membranes during labour, there is no clear evidence to suggest that active management of labour is of benefit to all labouring women. Balanced information on the risks and benefits of the individual components, as well as the 'package' of active management as a policy of care, should be fully discussed with women during the antenatal period to allow them time to make truly informed choices.

■ Recommendations for clinical practice in the light of currently available evidence

1. True informed consent should be encouraged by the provision to women of evidence-based information outlining the benefits and risks of care strategies that may be employed during labour. This should include information about the limits of technological aids.

2. Midwives should seek to assume an active role in ensuring the appropriateness of interventions such as active management policies and the use of technological aids such as fetal monitors. The research evidence to date has not shown them to be of indisputable benefit in improving health outcomes for women or fetuses.

3. Mechanisms for vigilant and continuous monitoring of current labour management policies should be put in place in order to ensure that the essence of the policy does not alter from the original protocol without there being appropriate multidisciplinary consultation and evaluation.

■ Practice check

- What are the rates in your unit for amniotomy, oxytocin augmentation, instrumental delivery and caesarean section?

- How do you define the onset of labour? How often is your definition the same as that of the women themselves?

- What is the longest duration of labour among women in your care? At what stage is intervention offered?

- Are women in your unit allowed to eat and drink while in labour if they wish?

- How involved are the women in your care in choices about the management of their own labour? Do you consult women before performing an amniotomy or setting up an oxytocin drip?

- What is your unit's policy on the use of continuous fetal monitoring?

- How confident do you feel about challenging unit policy if you feel it is not necessarily in the interests of a woman and/or her fetus?

■ References

Bonovich L 1990 Recognising the onset of labour. Journal of Obstetric, Gynecologic and Neonatal Nursing 19(2): 141–5

Boylan PC 1989 Active management of labour: results in Dublin, Houston, London, New Brunswick, Singapore and Valparaiso. Birth 16(3): 114–18

De Mott RK, Sandmire HF 1992 The Green Bay caesarean section study. The physician factor as a determinant of caesarean birth rates for failed labour. American Journal of Obstetrics and Gynecology June: 1799–807

Frigoletto F, Liebman E, Lang PHJM *et al* 1992 A controlled trial of a programme for the active management of labour. New England Journal of Medicine 326: 450–4

Garcia J, Corry M, MacDonald D, Elbourne D, Grant A 1985 Mothers' views of continuous electronic fetal heart monitoring and intermittent auscultation: a randomised controlled trial. Birth 12(2): 79–86

Hannah M, Ohlsson A, Fanne D *et al*, for the Term PROM Study Group 1996 Induction of labour compared with expectant management for preterm rupture of membranes at term. New England Journal of Medicine 334(16): 1005–10

Haverkamp AD, Thompson HE, McFee JG *et al* 1976 The evaluation of continuous fetal heart rate monitoring in high risk pregnancy. American Journal of Obstetrics and Gynecology 134(3): 310–20

Howell CJ 1995 Epidural vs non-epidural analgesia in labour. In Pregnancy and Childbirth Module of Cochrane Database of Systematic Reviews, disk issue 1. Available from BMJ Publishing Group, London

Inch S 1985 Management of the third stage of labour – another cascade of intervention. Midwifery 1(1): 114–22

Keirse MJNC 1995 Amniotomy plus early vs late oxytocic infusion for induction of labour. In Pregnancy and Childbirth Module of the Cochrane Database of Systematic Reviews, disk issue 2. Available from BMJ Publishing Group, London

Kelso IM, Parsons RJ, Lawrence GF 1978 An assessment of continuous fetal heart rate monitoring in labour: a randomised trial. American Journal of Obstetrics and Gynecology 131(5): 526–32

Lopez-Zeno JA, Peaceman AH, Adashek JA, Socol ML 1992 Commentaries: Failure to progress in the management of labour. British Journal of Obstetrics and Gynaecology 101: 1–3

MIDIRS/NHS Centre for Reviews and Dissemination 1996 Informed Choice leaflets. MIDIRS/NHS, Bristol and London

Mold JW, Stein HF 1986 Sounding board: The cascade effect in the clinical care of patients. New England Journal of Medicine 314(8): 512–14

Neilson J 1995 Electronic fetal monitoring plus scalp sampling vs intermittent auscultation in labour. In Pregnancy and Childbirth Module of Cochrane Database of Systematic Reviews, disk issue 2. Available from BMJ Publishing Group, London

O'Driscoll K 1993 Active management of labour, 3rd edn. WB Saunders, London

O'Driscoll K, Meagher D 1986 Active management of labour, 2nd edn. WB Saunders, London

O'Driscoll K, Jackson RJA, Gallagher J 1969 Prevention of prolonged labour. British Medical Journal 2: 447–80

Olah KS, Neilson JP 1994 Editorial: Failure to progress in the management of labour. British Journal of Obstetrics and Gynaecology 101(1): 1–3

Porreco R 1990 Meeting the challenges of the rising caesarean birth rate. Obstetrics and Gynecology 5: 133–6

Shearer E 1989 Commentaries: The caesarean section rate is 25% and rising. Why? What can be done about it? Birth 16(3): 119–20

Thornton JG, Lilford RJ 1994 Active management of labour: current knowledge and research issues. British Medical Journal 309: 366–9

Turnbull H, Laing S 1995 Select Committee on Intervention. In Childbirth Report, Legislative Assembly of Western Australia. State Law Publisher, Perth, WA p29

Chapter 5

Emergencies during labour: umbilical cord prolapse and inversion of the uterus

Maxine Wallis-Redworth

Any emergency during labour can be a frightening experience for both the woman and the attending midwife. There is the potential for maternal and fetal morbidity or mortality. The midwife is a key player in the prevention, prompt recognition and initiation of appropriate intervention to reduce any negative impact. In order to achieve this, the midwife needs to possess up to date knowledge and be able to discern the most appropriate management approach for the individual situations faced. Two such situations are umbilical cord prolapse and inversion of the uterus. The author's anecdotal inquiry has revealed variation in midwives' knowledge and expertise in dealing with the aforementioned emergencies. This inquiry has been important in shaping the approach to and content of the chapter.

■ It is assumed that you are already aware of the following:

- The anatomy of the reproductive tract;
- The anatomy of the umbilical cord;
- The physiology of labour, particularly the third stage of labour;
- Management of the third stage of labour;
- The risks of specific obstetric interventions, for example artificial rupture of the membranes;
- The features of obstetric shock.

■ Umbilical cord prolapse

☐ Definition

Umbilical cord prolapse is when a portion of the umbilical cord lies below or in front of the presenting part and the membranes have ruptured (Koonings *et al* 1990; Mesleh *et al* 1993). Distinction is made between overt cord prolapse, when the cord is at the level of or has passed through the cervix, and occult prolapse, when the cord may lie between the fetus and the uterine wall (Critchlow *et al* 1994).

Although there are cases documented prior to the onset of established labour, there is consensus that umbilical cord prolapse is more a phenomenon of the first stage of labour (Vago 1970; Chetty and Moodley 1980; Caspi *et al* 1983; Yla-Outinen *et al* 1985; Katz *et al* 1988; Koonings *et al* 1990; Critchlow *et al* 1994; Murphy and MacKenzie 1995).

☐ Incidence

The reported incidence varies considerably, for example 1 in 239 being given by Caspi *et al* (1983), 1 in 426 by Murphy and MacKenzie (1995) and 1 in 714 deliveries by Yla-Outinen *et al* (1985). All but one of the studies surveyed present retrospective data relating to one hospital only, the exception being a population-based case-control study based on births over 5 years within Washington state, USA (Critchlow *et al* 1994).

There is very little discussion on why such a variation in incidence is seen. In part, it may be due to the way in which cord prolapse is either classified or recorded. Many authors do not specify the nature of the records accessed, but it would appear that these vary in the amount of detail they contain. Critchlow *et al* (1994) used birth certificates but noted that the use of the full obstetric record could possibly have overcome the lack of detailed information. Equally, it may have to be accepted that the varying incidence reflects characteristics of the women whose labours were complicated by umbilical cord prolapse, as well as the varying intrapartum practices of the specific hospitals, such as the practice of rupture of the membranes in the early phase of the first stage of labour.

☐ Cause and associated factors

The basic cause of umbilical cord prolapse is the absence or instability of the presenting part in the pelvis. There are a number of situations that may prevent the presenting part from adequately filling the pelvis – malpresentations, multiple pregnancy, multiparity and preterm/low birthweight. Equally, obstetric procedures or interventions are strongly implicated (Levy *et al* 1984). Factors with a loose association with cord prolapse include a long umbilical cord (Cavanagh *et al* 1982), delivery in hospital (Levy *et al*

1984) and a maternal age of over 30 (Woo *et al* 1983). This last finding could be explained by a loose association between increasing parity and increasing maternal age. It must be remembered that, in many countries, the majority of babies, in particular those to women considered to be at high risk, are born in hospital, thus perhaps increasing the likelihood of cord prolapse occurring in hospital rather than at home.

☐ *Malpresentations*

In many studies, malpresentations of the fetus play a significant part in umbilical cord prolapse (Migliorini and Pepperell 1977; Caspi *et al* 1983; Woo *et al* 1983; Levy *et al* 1984; Yla-Outinen *et al* 1985; Katz *et al* 1988; Koonings *et al* 1990; Murphy & MacKenzie 1995). Breech presentations are the most commonly associated malpresentations and, where specifically identified, account for 10–16 per cent of cases of cord prolapse (Critchlow *et al* 1994; Yla-Outinen *et al* 1985). This, however, reflects the normal proportion of breech presentation compared with other types of malpresentation.

☐ *Multiple pregnancy*

Multiple pregnancy also appears to increase the risk of umbilical cord prolapse (Levy *et al* 1984; Koonings *et al* 1990). The number of fetuses being referred to in multiple pregnancy is not always obvious, but some studies specifically refer to twins (Yla-Outinen *et al* 1985; Critchlow *et al* 1994; Murphy & MacKenzie 1995). There is consensus that the second twin is more likely to be affected (Critchlow *et al* 1994; Murphy & MacKenzie 1995), probably because of the higher incidence of malpresentation (Critchlow *et al* 1994). No reports identify both fetuses being affected concurrently.

☐ *Multiparity*

The association between umbilical cord prolapse and multiparity is frequently noted, but possible underlying reasons for this are infrequently discussed (Clark *et al* 1968; Levy *et al* 1984; Yla-Outinen *et al* 1985; Koonings *et al* 1990; Critchlow *et al* 1994; Ritchie 1995). As many as 80 per cent of cases occur in multiparous women, especially those of higher parity (Clark *et al* 1968; Murphy & MacKenzie 1995; Ritchie 1995). Two possible reasons for this association are the increased possibility of a weakened lower uterine segment and loss of abdominal muscle tone in multiparous women, and the increased incidence of non-engagement of the presenting part until labour is well established (Clark *et al* 1968; Ritchie 1995).

☐ *Preterm/low birthweight*

A birthweight of below 2500 g is associated with up to one third of cases of umbilical cord prolapse (Woo *et al* 1983; Levy *et al* 1984; Yla-Outinen *et al* 1985; Koonings *et al* 1990; Critchlow *et al* 1994; Murphy & MacKenzie 1995). There is a definite association between preterm birth and malpresentation (Clark *et al* 1968). When cord prolapse occurs, low birthweight babies are noted to have a significantly higher perinatal mortality rate than other babies. Yla-Outinen *et al* (1985) showed a gross perinatal mortality rate of 16.2 per cent that decreased to 3.6 per cent when only babies weighing over 2500 g were considered.

☐ *Obstetric interventions*

A number of studies show an association between artificial rupture of the membranes and cord prolapse (Mesleh *et al* 1993; Murphy & MacKenzie 1995), while other researchers show a less significant or nil association (Levy *et al* 1984; Yla-Outinen *et al* 1985).

In Murphy and MacKenzie's study, over 50 per cent of cord prolapses occurred within the first 5 minutes after membrane rupture. It is not clear whether this is only true of artificial rupture of the membranes or of all cases of ruptured membranes. At the time of diagnosis, 66 per cent of cases were recorded as having a high presenting part, but there is no comment on whether the high presenting part had been noted prior to the cord prolapse. Cord prolapse is more likely to occur if the stability of the presenting part is not correctly assessed prior to artificial rupture of the membranes (Barrett 1991). So it could be concluded that it may not be the procedure of artificial rupture of membranes *per se* that increases the risk of cord prolapse but the lack of recognition of instability of the presenting part. Displacement upwards of an unstable presenting part during vaginal examination may account for some cases of cord prolapse following spontaneous rupture of the membranes; equally, displacement may occur during the application of a fetal scalp electrode or while undertaking fetal blood sampling (Levy *et al* 1984). In such situations, awareness of the possibility of such an 'accident' should not only reduce its occurrence, but also lead to prompt diagnosis.

☐ Diagnosis

Definitive diagnosis is usually by vaginal examination or visualisation. Perinatal mortality is lower when diagnosis is made by vaginal examination (Woo *et al* 1983). This could be because the prolapse–to–diagnosis interval is shorter and therefore prompt intervention can be initiated. In more recent times, the use of cardiotocography monitoring has facilitated earlier recognition of the consequence of cord prolapse – cord compression (Caspi *et al* 1983). Two specific features – variable deceleration and prolonged deceleration – are considered to be reliable signs of cord compression and are best identified using cardiotocography (Koonings *et al* 1990; Gibb & Arulkumaran 1992; Murphy & MacKenzie 1995).

Appropriate utilisation of this technology will facilitate not only earlier diagnosis, but also earlier intervention aimed at reducing the perinatal mortality and morbidity. In units where the availability of cardiotocography monitors is limited, it is suggested that they are used for labours in which actual or potential risk factors have been identified (Haverkamp 1991; MacDonald 1991).

Once cord prolapse has been identified, there is a need for further information, namely the degree of cervical dilatation and the fetal condition. Cervical dilatation is a central factor in determining management (Vago 1970). With regard to the assessment of fetal condition, Ritchie (1995) advocates performing a vaginal examination and auscultating the fetal heart whenever the membranes rupture. Fetal condition can be assessed during vaginal examination by the presence or absence of pulsation in the cord, although this is not considered to be a precise indicator (Migliorini & Pepperell 1977; Driscoll *et al* 1987). Auscultation of the fetal heart is a priority. In the absence of a pulsating cord and audible fetal heart sounds, the use of real-time ultrasound is advocated to confirm the diagnosis of fetal death (Driscoll *et al* 1987). This course of action, although time consuming, is considered critical by some practitioners in producing an holistic assessment and promoting positive perinatal outcomes (Griese & Prickett 1993). While mortality may be avoided, there must be a question of the degree of morbidity being sustained when a fetus without a pulsating cord or audible fetal heart sounds is delivered and subsequently resuscitated. Indeed, Driscoll *et al* (1987) acknowledge such concerns. Of two such cases reported by them in which ultrasound was used, survival in one instance may be attributed to the baby being born at term following a prompt caesarean section and of an appropriate birthweight. The interrelation of multiple factors makes it extremely difficult to determine which, if any, is the most significant. In view of the extremely small number of cases using such an approach, caution must be exercised in advocating a more widespread use of ultrasound in the absence of pulsation in the umbilical cord and audible fetal heart sounds.

☐ Management

There is a consensus that prompt and correct diagnosis followed by decisive intervention are the major contributors to the successful management of cord prolapse (Katz *et al* 1988; Griese & Prickett 1993). Yla-Outinen *et al* (1985) in Finland attributed a reduction in perinatal mortality over a 19-year period to an increase in the rate of caesarean section, advances in the antenatal diagnosis of malpresentation and advances in neonatal intensive care.

Current management of diagnosed or suspected umbilical cord prolapse focuses on efforts to relieve pressure of the presenting part on the umbilical cord while preparations are made for immediate delivery.

☐ *Relief of pressure on the umbilical cord*

This can be achieved in several ways:

● Manual elevation of the presenting part;

● Maternal positioning;

● Bladder filling.

Manual elevation of the presenting part

Manual elevation is most commonly achieved by the vaginal route, aiming to elevate the presenting part above the pelvic brim and thus relieving cord compression. Vago (1970) claims that it is a highly effective measure but provides no evidence to support this. Whether or not it is a highly effective measure, it has certain drawbacks. The woman can find it physically uncomfortable and psychologically embarrassing, and, if it has to be continued for any length of time, the clinician in attendance can tire (Chetty & Moodley 1980), with the potential for a less effective relief of cord compression. A possible alternative, not considered within the literature, is that of elevation of the presenting part per abdomen. While such an approach may reduce embarrassment for the woman, in itself an important consideration, the top priority should be given to reducing the risk for the fetus.

Maternal positioning

The aim is to place the woman in a position that encourages the fetus to be displaced towards the fundus; thus the fundus needs to be at a lower level than the cervix. This can be achieved by placing the woman in either the Trendelenburg, Sims or knee–chest position (Chetty & Moodley 1980; Caspi *et al* 1983). These positions may be combined with manual elevation of the presenting part.

The Trendelenburg position can be uncomfortable for any woman prone to supine hypotension, while the knee–chest position may be embarrassing for the woman and may impede preparation for delivery (Chetty & Moodley 1980). The knee–chest position may also be difficult to assume and maintain during active labour. While the Trendelenburg position can be uncomfortable, it is still the position most frequently recommended (Cavanagh *et al* 1982; Oxorn 1986).

Bladder filling

This is a technique practised outside the UK. It was first described by Vago (1970) as a means of relieving cord compression by preventing descent of the presenting part. Following diagnosis, a no. 16 Foley catheter is inserted into the bladder and approximately 500 ml of normal saline quickly introduced. The balloon is then inflated and the catheter clamped. Vago (1970) also noted that a distended bladder led to a decline in uterine activity. Women may complain of some discomfort as a result of the rapid distension of the bladder (Griese & Prickett 1993). The exact amount of fluid needed appears to vary, the object being a presenting part that has been elevated by a full bladder. Such an elevation can be confirmed by abdominal palpation and the place at which the fetal heart is auscultated.

Various authors (Chetty & Moodley 1980; Caspi *et al* 1983) have used this technique as an interim means while awaiting caesarean section or to achieve the safe transportation of the woman to a more appropriate unit prior to delivery. Chetty and Moodley (1980) reported 24 cases using bladder filling with no perinatal mortality despite a mean diagnosis-to-delivery interval of 69 minutes. In eight cases, the diagnosis-to-delivery interval was greater than 80 minutes. Twenty-one of the babies had Apgar scores of 9 or 10 at 1 minute, the minimum score being 6. Thus the vast majority showed no adverse effects from the delay. While the mode of delivery is not explicit, there is an assumption of caesarean section. Caspi *et al* (1983) reported 127 cases in which the fetus was alive at the time of diagnosis of overt cord prolapse. There were no perinatal deaths among the 88 cases managed by caesarean section. Griese and Prickett (1993) described a case where, within 10 minutes of bladder filling, fetal heart rate recordings were reactive. This, however, is an isolated case report.

☐ *Type of delivery and outcome*

Unless the cervix is fully dilated and it is judged that a vaginal delivery can be achieved quickly, there is universal agreement that caesarean section is the optimal mode of delivery in order to improve neonatal outcome. Caesarean section rates in the region of 70–96 per cent for cases of cord prolapse are reported (Koonings *et al* 1990; Critchlow *et al* 1994; Murphy & MacKenzie 1995). These statistics are not surprising given that the largest proportion of cases diagnosed during the first stage of labour lead to caesarean section as the preferred mode of delivery to achieve optimal neonatal outcome. The findings of Critchlow *et al* (1994) suggest that the risks of asphyxia, low Apgar scores and subsequent mortality are decreased by caesarean section when compared with vaginal deliveries.

High caesarean section rates generally correlate with low perinatal mortality, although Caspi *et al* (1983) do not claim that their low rate is attributable only to caesarean section but also to bladder filling and, importantly, cardiotocography monitoring, which allows the early recognition of the resultant cord compression. They state that this enables prompt and accurate diagnosis and the appropriate intervention. Koonings *et al* (1990) claim that any decrease in medical intervention will lead to an increase in perinatal mortality rate, although it is not clear what they classify as medical intervention.

, Caspi *et al* (1983) provide a note of caution, suggesting that section should not be the universal treatment since the procedure ,sociated with a significant perinatal mortality.

■ Recommendations for clinical practice in the light of currently available evidence

1. Initial assessment at the beginning of intrapartum care should identify actual or potential risk factors for umbilical cord prolapse, and these should be clearly documented.

2. A protocol for the early recognition of umbilical cord prolapse is necessary to promote a good fetal/neonatal outcome. This protocol should promote the use of abdominal examination following actual or suspected rupture of the membranes in order that situations such as malpresentation and non-engagement of the presenting part are identified quickly and that fetal wellbeing is established at the earliest possible time.

3. Artificial rupture of the membranes should not be undertaken until risk factors such as malpresentation and a non-engaged presenting part are excluded.

4. Each maternity unit should identify the specific measures to be used to achieve elevation of the presenting part in the event of cord prolapse.

5. Each maternity unit should have in place audit processes to monitor the outcomes of the management of umbilical cord prolapse.

■ Practice check

● Are you aware of the incidence of umbilical cord prolapse in your unit? Can you identify any apparent link between its occurrence and any particular predisposing factors?

● Following vaginal examination and after rupture of the membranes, do you record the fetal heart rate?

● Are you aware of the guidelines, in your unit, for dealing with emergencies such as umbilical cord prolapse?

● What is the diagnosis-to-delivery interval in your unit?

■ Inversion of the uterus

□ Definition

Uterine inversion is best described as the uterus being turned inside out (O'Sullivan 1945; Bell *et al* 1953; Lago 1991), this usually being a rapid event. It is a complication generally associated with the third stage of labour, mostly occurring during or soon after its completion (Kitchin *et al* 1975; Moretti & Sibai 1990; Lago 1991).

Various classifications are to be found within the literature, which spans the last 65 years. The classifications are based on the position of the inverted uterine fundus or the time elapsing between delivery and diagnosis of the inversion.

The most common classification identifies three types of inversion related to the position of the inverted fundus: first degree, in which the fundus remains within the uterine cavity; second degree, in which the fundus passes through the cervix into the vagina; and third degree, with the uterus completely turned inside out and lying in the vagina or even outside the vulva (Donald 1979; Lago 1991).

The majority of cases of uterine inversion occur within 24 hours of delivery and are classified as acute, while subacute inversion is classified as that occurring within the first month after delivery (Wendel & Cox 1995).

□ Incidence

Estimates of incidence vary from 1:20 000 (Bunke & Hofmeister 1965) to between 1:1700 and 1:2500 (Kitchin *et al* 1975; Platt & Druzin 1981; Brar *et al* 1989; Zahn & Yeomans 1990). It is not always clear whether the reported incidence involves all categories of the classification given above.

The incidence of uterine inversion is noted to be relatively unchanged over time (Platt & Druzin 1981; Brar *et al* 1989). Those authors who note an apparent increase in the incidence of uterine inversion cannot offer any reasons (Kitchin *et al* 1975; Shah-Hosseini & Evrard 1989).

There appears to be some consensus that uterine inversion generally occurs after a term pregnancy (Platt & Druzin 1981; Wendel & Cox 1995), but this may merely reflect the total proportion of vaginal deliveries occurring at this stage of pregnancy and the larger proportion of caesarean deliveries in preterm infants.

□ Cause

The actual cause of uterine inversion remains somewhat uncertain, although there is a widely held view that uterine inversion is the result of mismanagement of the third stage of labour (Bunke & Hofmeister 1965; Donald 1979;

Rauff 1989; Moretti & Sibai 1990). This is, however, contested
~~~~er of authors (Das 1940; Kitchin *et al* 1975; Watson *et al* 1980;
~~~~1989; Shah-Hosseini & Evrard 1989). The particular actions and
~~~~~at are considered to contribute to the risk of uterine inversion
incl. mismanagement of the third stage of labour as a result of excessive
traction on the umbilical cord, especially before placental separation, and
pressure on the fundus in an attempt to expel the placenta or clots from the
uterine cavity (Donald 1979). Inversion will only occur in the presence of
cervical dilatation and of relaxation of part of the uterine body (Bell *et al*
1953; Ratnam & Rauff 1989). It will not occur if the uterus is contracted
and retracted (Beazley 1995).

Watson *et al* (1980) suggest that, apart from a previous history of
inversion and an ultrasonically located fundal placenta, there is no single
predisposing factor that acts as a warning for uterine inversion. The review
by Das (1940) identified that approximately 75 per cent of cases had a
completely or partially adherent fundal placenta. A fundally located placenta
in the presence of uterine atony would appear to increase the risk of uterine
inversion if inappropriate action, such as cord traction or fundal pressure to
expel the placenta, were taken by the birth attendant (Donald 1979).

Other factors that have been suggested to be associated with uterine
inversion include primiparity (Das 1940; Brar *et al* 1989; Shah-Hosseini &
Evrard 1989) and large babies (Brar *et al* 1989). The evidence for such
association is not well addressed.

While inversion can be associated with specific intrapartum events; it
is estimated that 13–40 per cent of cases occur spontaneously; it is
postulated that the basis for spontaneous inversion lies within the uterus,
for example fundal implantation of the placenta (Das 1940; Bell *et al*
1953; Kitchin *et al* 1975; Ratnam & Rauff 1989). Attributing the cause to
mismanagement of the third stage of labour should perhaps be avoided
unless specific evidence exists.

☐ Diagnosis

This relies on observation of the mother's condition and a knowledge of
the classification of uterine inversion. Prompt recognition is vital to facilitate swift replacement before the cervix contracts. Presenting signs and
symptoms can easily lead to an incomplete diagnosis, such as postpartum
haemorrhage, being made. Any newly delivered mother who has had a
postpartum haemorrhage, and whose shock is not responding as anticipated to treatment, needs to be examined vaginally to rule out uterine
inversion. First and second degrees of inversion may not easily be identified, whereas third degree inversion, while uncommon, is unlikely to be
missed (Donald 1979).

☐ Signs

These are dependent on the degree of the inversion. Haemorrhage is the cardinal sign, with a wide variation in blood loss that appears to be related to the time lapse since inversion (Watson *et al* 1980). Shock is also an accompanying feature.

However, the shock may be out of proportion to the amount of blood loss. The shock has neurogenic and hypovolaemic elements; the first is attributed to traction on intra-abdominal structures while the latter is caused by the volume of blood loss (Moretti & Sibai 1990). Abdominal examination may demonstrate two cardinal uterine signs: apparent absence of the fundus and palpable cupping in the fundal area (Moretti & Sibai 1990).

☐ Management

The aim of management is to prevent maternal mortality and morbidity. Kitchin *et al* (1975) claim that zero mortality is possible because of the availability of blood transfusion, antibiotics and oxytocics. Such availability, however, is not universal. Where mortality exists, it would appear to be due to a delay in diagnosis (Olah & Fishwick 1995).

Correct management of the third stage of labour is the most important measure to prevent uterine inversion (Kitchin *et al* 1975; Ratnam & Rauff 1989). It would seem that future efforts to reduce maternal mortality need to be focused not only on prevention, but also on prompt diagnosis and the initiation of a range of interventions deemed appropriate for the individual mother (Lee *et al* 1978). This emphasis on prevention is important not least because individual practitioners are unlikely to have a wealth of personal experience in the recognition and treatment of uterine inversion.

Midwifery action after the diagnosis of an actual or suspected case of uterine inversion includes raising the foot of the bed, calling for medical aid, correcting the accompanying shock using defined protocols and preparing for correction of the inversion (Towler & Butler-Manuel 1975; Sleep 1993).

In the absence of medical aid, it may be reasonable for the midwife to attempt immediate replacement of the inversion; should this be unsuccessful, further efforts to do so should not be made by the attending midwife, who has fulfilled the remit of emergency action as permitted in the Midwife's Code of Practice Section 5.7 (UKCC 1994).

☐ *Replacement of the uterus*

Prompt replacement overcomes the problems of the fundus becoming bulkier as a result of the development of oedema and cervical constriction (Lee *et al* 1978). Rapid reduction of the inversion may be achieved vaginally.

Using the fingertips, upwards pressure towards the umbilicus is applied to the area adjacent to the cervix (Bell *et al* 1953; Lago 1991; Olah & Fishwick 1995). Such a technique promotes the principle of 'last out, first back' and attempts to prevent multiple thicknesses of the myometrium being present at the level of the cervical ring, thus impeding replacement (Kitchin *et al* 1975; Platt & Druzin 1981; Lago 1991).

Replacement of the uterus prior to removal of the placenta is widely advocated on the grounds that an intact placenta reduces the risk of haemorrhage and a deepening of shock (Kitchin *et al* 1975; Brar *et al* 1989; Moretti & Sibai 1990), a change in practice over the last 50 years. Only if the placenta is already separating or its bulk makes replacement difficult is the placenta removed (Donald 1979).

If manual repositioning is unsuccessful, the technique universally advocated to replace the inverted uterus involves hydrostatic pressure. O'Sullivan (1945) discovered the technique by chance while giving an antiseptic douche before using the accepted treatment of the day. O'Sullivan's technique involves increasing intravaginal pressure by blocking the introitus of the vagina with the operator's wrist or lower forearm. The operator or assistant may need to ensure that the labia are gathered around the forearm to achieve appropriate blockage. Large volumes (up to 6 litres) of warm normal saline are infused via an intravenous giving set to distend the vagina. The fluid causes an increase of pressure, which pushes the inverted uterus upwards and relieves any cervical constriction by stretching the four vaginal fornices (Olah & Fishwick 1995). The important contraindication of a ruptured uterus should be excluded first (Ratnam & Rauff 1989). Marked cervical constriction may prevent the successful use of O'Sullivan's technique (Donald 1979), but this may be overcome using general anaesthesia. In the USA during the 1980s, tocolytic drugs such as terbutaline sulphate became popular to overcome difficult or unsuccessful manual repositioning (Kovacs & DeVore 1984; Catanzarite *et al* 1986; Brar *et al* 1989). The particular properties of these drugs were preferred to those of general anaesthesia.

Once the uterus is successfully repositioned, uterine contraction needs to be established to avoid the risk of reinversion, which may occur within hours or days (Catanzarite *et al* 1986). Intravenous oxytocics are the favoured means (Watson *et al* 1980; Kovacs & DeVore 1984; Brar *et al* 1989; Moretti & Sibai 1990), but prostaglandins have also been utilised, both intramuscularly and directly injected into either the cervix or myometrium (Thiery and Delbeke 1985; Brar *et al* 1989). Despite reported success with prostaglandins, using oxytocics appears to be the prevailing practice.

Replacing the inverted uterus may predispose to infection. The use of prophylactic antibiotics is controversial, with no benefit in terms of a reduction of postpartum febrile morbidity being demonstrated in a number of studies (Kitchin *et al* 1975; Watson *et al* 1980; Platt & Druzin 1981). Despite the urgency in undertaking replacement of the inverted uterus, it cannot be stressed enough that proper aseptic technique is of paramount importance for the prevention of infection.

■ Recommendations for clinical practice in the light of currently available evidence

1. Each midwife needs to be aware of and alert to predisposing factors, for example a fundal placenta or a previous uterine inversion.

2. Each unit should have a clear and agreed protocol for the active management of the third stage of labour when such management is requested or deemed appropriate.

3. The prompt recognition of uterine inversion will facilitate the earliest possible replacement of the uterus and the correction of shock.

4. All midwives must know the unit protocol for the emergency management of an inverted uterus in the absence of medical aid.

■ Practice check

● Do you check each woman's history for factors predisposing to uterine inversion?

● Does your unit have an agreed protocol for the management of uterine inversion?

● Are you aware of the steps needed promptly to replace an inverted uterus in the absence of medical aid?

■ References

Barrett JM 1991 Funic reduction for the management of umbilical cord prolapse. American Journal of Obstetrics and Gynecology 165(3): 654-7

Beazley JM 1995 Complications of the third stage of labour. In Whitfield CR (ed.) Dewhurst's Textbook of obstetrics and gynaecology for postgraduates, 5th edn. Blackwell Science, Oxford, Ch 25, pp368–76

Bell JE, Wilson GF, Wilson LA 1953 Puerperal inversion of the uterus. American Journal of Obstetrics and Gynecology 66(4): 767–80

Brar HS, Greenspoon JS, Platt LD, Paul RH 1989 Acute puerperal uterine inversion – new approaches to management. Journal of Reproductive Medicine 34(2): 173–7

Bunke JW, Hofmeister FJC 1965 Uterine inversion – obstetrical entity or oddity. American Journal of Obstetrics and Gynecology 91(7): 934–9

Caspi E, Lotan Y, Schreyer P 1983 Prolapse of the cord: reduction of perinatal mortality by bladder instillation and cesarean section. Israel Journal of Medical Sciences 19: 541–5

Catanzarite VA, Moffitt KD, Baker ML, Awadalla SG, Argubrigh KF, Perkins RP 1986 New approaches to the management of acute puerperal uterine inversion. Obstetrics and Gynecology 68(3) (supplement): 7S–10S

Cavanagh HD, Woods RE, O'Connor TCF, Knuppel RA 1982 Obstetric emergencies, 3rd edn. Harper & Row, Philadelphia

Chetty RM, Moodley J 1980 Umbilical cord prolapse. South African Medical Journal 57: 128–9

Clark DO, Copeland W, Ullery JC 1968 Prolapse of the umbilical cord. American Journal of Obstetrics and Gynecology 101(1): 84–90

Critchlow CW, Leet TL, Benedetti TJ, Daling JR 1994 Risk factors and infant outcomes associated with umbilical cord prolapse: a population-based case-control study among births in Washington state. American Journal of Obstetrics and Gynecology 170(2): 613–18

Das P 1940 Inversion of the uterus. Journal of Obstetrics and Gynaecology of the British Empire 47: 525–48

Donald I 1979 Practical obstetric problems, 5th edn. Lloyd-Luke, London, p 804–11

Driscoll JA, Sadan O, Van Gelderen CJ, Holloway GA 1987 Cord prolapse: can we save more babies? Case reports. British Journal of Obstetrics and Gynaecology 94: 594–5

Gibb D, Arulkumaran S 1992 Fetal monitoring in practice. Butterworth Heinemann, Oxford, Ch 4, pp22–39

Griese ME, Prickett SA 1993 Nursing management of umbilical cord prolapse. Journal of Obstetric, Gynecologic and Neonatal Nursing 22(4): 311–15

Haverkamp A 1991 Fetal monitoring in high-risk labour. In Spencer J (ed.) Fetal monitoring – physiology and techniques of antenatal and intrapartum assessment. Oxford University Press, Oxford, Ch 36, pp207–10

Katz Z, Shoham Z, Lancet M, Blickstein I, Mogilner BM, Zalel Y 1988 Management of labour with umbilical cord prolapse: a 5-year study. Obstetrics and Gynecology 72: 278–81

Kitchin JD, Thiagarajah S, May HV, Thornton WN 1975 Puerperal inversion of the uterus. American Journal of Obstetrics and Gynecology 123(1): 51–8

Koonings PP, Paul RH, Campbell K 1990 Umbilical cord prolapse: a contemporary look. Journal of Reproductive Medicine 35: 690–2

Kovacs BW, DeVore GR 1984 Management of acute and subacute puerperal uterine inversion with terbutaline sulfate. American Journal of Obstetrics and Gynecology 150(6): 784–86

Lago JD 1991 Presentation of acute uterine inversion in the emergency department. American Journal of Emergency Medicine 9(3): 239–42

Lee WK, Baggish MS, Lashgari M 1978 Acute inversion of the uterus. Obstetrics and Gynecology 51: 144

Levy H, Meier PR, Makowski EL 1984 Umbilical cord prolapse. Obstetrics and Gynecology 64: 499–502

MacDonald D 1991 Fetal monitoring in normal labour. In Spencer J (ed.) Fetal monitoring – physiology and techniques of antenatal and intrapartum assessment. Oxford University Press, Oxford, Ch 35, pp202–6

Mesleh R, Sultan M, Sabagh T, Algwiser A 1993 Umbilical cord prolapse. Journal of Obstetrics and Gynecology 13(1): 24–8

Migliorini GD, Pepperell RJ 1977 Prolapse of the umbilical cord: a study of 69 cases. Medical Journal of Australia 2: 522–4

Moretti ML, Sibai BM 1990 Peripartum emergencies. In Benrubi GI (ed.) Contemporary issues in emergency medicine – obstetric emergencies. Churchill Livingstone, New York

Murphy D, Mackenzie I 1995 The mortality and morbidity associated with umbilical cord prolapse. British Journal of Obstetrics and Gynaecology 102(10): 826–30

Olah KS, Fishwick K 1995 Management of acute uterine inversion. British Journal of Midwifery 3(2): 83–7

O'Sullivan JV 1945 Acute inversion of the uterus. British Medical Journal ii: 282–3

Oxorn H 1986 Human labour and birth, 5th edn. Appleton-Century-Crofts, Norwalk, CT, Ch 21, pp284–9

Platt LD, Druzin ML 1981 Acute puerperal inversion of the uterus. American Journal of Obstetrics and Gynecology 141(2): 187–90

Ratnam S, Rauff M 1989 Postpartum haemorrhage and abnormalities of the third stage of labour. In Turnbull A, Chamberlain G (eds) Obstetrics. Churchill Livingstone, Edinburgh, Ch 59, pp867–76

Ritchie JWK 1995 Malpositions of the occiput and malpresentations. In Whitfield CR (ed.) Dewhurst's Textbook of obstetrics and gynaecology for postgraduates, 5th edn. Blackwell Science, Oxford, Ch 24, pp346–67

Shah-Hosseini R, Evrard JR 1989 Puerperal uterine inversion. Obstetrics and Gynecology 73(4): 567–70

Sleep J 1993 Complications of the third stage of labour. In Bennett VR, Brown LK (eds) Myles Textbook for midwives, 12th edn. Churchill Livingstone, Edinburgh, Ch 29, pp462–76

Thiery M, Delbeke L 1985 Acute puerperal uterine inversion: two-step management with a B-mimetic and a prostaglandin. American Journal of Obstetrics and Gynecology 153(8): 891–2

Towler J, Butler-Manuel R 1975 Modern obstetrics for student midwives. Lloyd-Luke, London, pp495–6

United Kingdom Central Council for Nursing, Midwifery and Heath Visiting 1994 A midwife's code of practice. UKCC, London

Vago T 1970 Prolapse of the umbilical cord: a method of management. American Journal of Obstetrics and Gynecology 107: 967–9

Watson P, Besch N, Bowes WA 1980 Management of acute and subacute puerperal inversion of the uterus. Obstetrics and Gynecology 55(1): 12–16

Wendel PJ, Cox SM 1995 Emergent obstetric management of uterine inversion. Obstetrics and Gynecology Clinics of North America 22(2): 261–74

Woo JS, Ngan YS, Ma HK 1983 Prolapse and presentation of the umbilical cord. Australian and New Zealand Journal of Obstetrics and Gynaecology 23: 142–5

Yla-Outinen A, Heinonen, PK, Tuimala, R 1985 Predisposing and risk factors of umbilical cord prolapse. Acta Obstetrica et Gynecologica Scandinavica 64: 567–70

Zahn CM, Yeomans ER 1990 Postpartum hemorrhage: placenta acreta, uterine inversion, and puerperal hematomas. Clinical Obstetrics and Gynecology 33(3): 422–31

■ Further reading

Koonings PP, Paul RH, Campbell K 1990 Umbilical cord prolapse: a contemporary look. Journal of Reproductive Medicine 35: 690–2

Lago JD 1991 Presentation of acute uterine inversion in the emergency department. American Journal of Emergency Medicine 9(3): 239–42

Wendel PJ, Cox SM 1995 Emergent obstetric management of uterine inversion. Obstetrics and Gynecology Clinics of North America 22(2): 261–74

Chapter 6

Diabetes mellitus in pregnancy

Tansy M Cheston

An article published in 1882, presenting a compiled case series of pregnancies complicated by diabetes reported in the world literature, found only 22 pregnancies in 15 diabetic women. Thirteen fetal deaths occured in 19 pregnancies, and nine of the women died within 1 year of the pregnancy (Duncan 1882). Few women with diabetes became pregnant until the discovery of insulin, as most patients died just 1 or 2 years after the onset of this illness. Before the discovery of insulin in 1923, those able to conceive had less than a 50 per cent chance of having a live child (Maresh & Beard 1995). The recognition that diabetes results in a disturbance of the environment of the fetus that may seriously interfere with organogenesis and development has led to the acknowledgement that normoglycaemia is an important objective in diabetic control.

Diabetes, which occurs in approximately 4 per 1000 pregnancies, is the most common pre-existing medical disorder complicating pregnancy in the UK (St Vincent Joint Task Force for Diabetes 1995, reported in Jardine Brown *et al* 1996). It is a high-risk state for both the woman and her fetus because of the increased risks of congenital malformation, miscarriage, ketoacidosis, pre-eclampsia, preterm labour, polyhydramnios, maternal infection, late intrauterine death, neonatal respiratory distress syndrome and jaundice. In addition, a significant deterioration of diabetic retinal and renal disease may occur, particularly in those women with a long history of poor diabetic control.

This chapter will consider research-based information on the maternal complications associated with diabetes mellitus and the effects that can occur in the fetus. It will aim to discuss current methods of diagnosing gestational diabetes, and introduce the findings of the 1995 St Vincent Declaration (Jardine Brown *et al* 1996) and how they should affect our management of the diabetic woman, preconceptually, antenatally and postpartum. The topics will be covered in the following order:

- Maternal complications: preconceptual care, retinopathy, renal and vascular complications, diabetic nephropathy and autonomic neuropathy;

- Pregnancy complications: preterm labour, hypoglycaemia and hyperglycaemia;

- Fetal complications: spontaneous miscarriage, congenital malformations, unexplained fetal death in utero and macrosomia;

- Neonatal complications: respiratory dysfunction, hypoglycaemia, and polycythaemia and jaundice;

- Gestational diabetes: predisposing factors, physiology and pathophysiology, and definition.

■ It is assumed that you are already aware of the following:

- The changes in glucose metabolism during pregnancy;

- The physiology of diabetes mellitus;

- Routine antenatal care.

■ The St Vincent Declaration

A Task Force was established in 1992 jointly by the Department of Health (DoH) and the British Diabetic Association to advise on the implementation of the St Vincent Declaration, which was the outcome of a meeting held in St Vincent in northern Italy in October 1989. It formulated a series of recommendations including both general goals and specific targets for improvement in the health and betterment of the lives of those with diabetes, and it urged the commitment of European nations to their fulfilment.

The issue of pregnancy and neonatal care was addressed by a subgroup chaired by Mr Michael Gillmer (a consultant obstetrician at the John Radcliffe Women's Centre in Oxford, UK). The group defined two priorities: first, targeting women with diabetes with preconceptual counselling, and second, promoting early referral for specialist care. The need for pregnancy care, labour and the delivery of women with diabetes to be undertaken only in specialised units was highlighted, as management by professional staff with training and experience in diabetes care was considered to secure optimal outcome. A screening procedure for gestational diabetes and the implementation of appropriate management was required. The main aim of the St Vincent Declaration was to 'achieve pregnancy outcome in diabetic women that approximates to that of non-diabetic women'.

In order to identify the facilities that are currently available for the care of pregnant diabetic women and to clarify the attitudes of physicians and obstetricians to their management, an extensive postal survey was undertaken between December 1993 and January 1994 by the Pregnancy and Neonatal Care Group of the Task Force. The replies formed the basis of the recommendations made for the care of the diabetic woman (Jardine Brown *et al* 1996).

The following section will review established diabetes mellitus and gestational diabetes, and then discuss the findings of the Pregnancy and Neonatal Group in the light of current recommendations for the care of women with diabetes in pregnancy.

■ Established diabetes mellitus

This is a term used to describe the state when diabetes is known to have been present before pregnancy. The vast majority of these women will have type 1, that is, insulin-dependent, diabetes mellitus (IDDM); the remainder will have type 2, non-insulin-dependent, diabetes mellitus (NIDDM).

☐ Maternal complications

☐ *Preconceptual care*

Extensive evidence has shown that an optimal outcome can be achieved in an insulin-dependent diabetic pregnancy if good glucose control is achieved before and during pregnancy (Lowy *et al* 1986). This requires pre-pregnancy counselling, including good contraceptive and dietary advice, together with early antenatal care by physicians, midwives and nurses, combined with careful obstetric surveillance and neonatal support.

To be effective, pre-pregnancy care must be commenced well before a diabetic woman considers having a family. Teenage girls must be warned of the risks of an unplanned pregnancy. All diabetic women considering conception should be made aware that their glucose control must be optimal before conceiving, thus reducing the risk of fetal congenital malformations. Attention should be paid to general health, contraception and good metabolic control, subjects which can be discussed by physicians, GPs, midwives and health visitors. The question of specific pre-pregnancy clinics is controversial, some health professionals arguing that easy access to a knowledgeable person (physician or obstetrician, specialist midwife or nurse) is more important (Drury & Doddridge 1992).

The major objective is to ensure that good diabetic control is maintained at the time of conception and embryogenesis. Those counselled before pregnancy were found to have lower long-term glucose concentrations in the blood (Steel *et al* 1990), lower glucose values in the first trimester and fewer congenital malformations among their babies (Fuhrmann *et al* 1983).

Preconceptual care allows time for women with type 2 diabetes mellitus to transfer from oral hypoglycaemic agents to insulin. Apart from the possible problems of transplacental drug passage and teratogenicity, the major reason for changing to insulin is the ability to maintain tighter control of glucose levels.

The St Vincent Declaration (Pregnancy and Neonatal Care Group) suggested that, as GPs provide most contraceptive services, they should be aware of the need for preconceptual counselling. Early referral, social support, continued prescribing of insulin, postnatal care and contraceptive advice should be provided by the GP and the primary health care team (Jardine Brown *et al* 1996).

☐ Retinopathy

Retinopathy should not be regarded as a contraindication to pregnancy. Almost all women will have background retinopathy after about 15 years of diabetes. Any retinopathy needs to be assessed and treated before pregnancy. Proliferative retinopathy can appear with further time, and, during the 9 months of pregnancy, new cases may arise (Dibble *et al* 1982). Provided that proliferative retinopathy (whether new or pre-existing) is actively treated, there appears to be no deterioration in visual acuity after pregnancy.

Background retinopathy may appear to deteriorate during pregnancy through impaired diabetic control, leading to an ischaemic retinopathy (Forrester *et al* 1989). Eye examinations should take place during pregnancy, and laser treatment can be undertaken if required.

☐ Renal and vascular complications

Fortunately, only a small proportion of diabetic women embarking on a pregnancy suffer from these complications; however, their problems require special consideration.

Diabetic nephropathy

The condition is manifested by increasing proteinuria, hypertension and fluid retention, all with or without evidence of decreasing renal function. This may worsen in pregnancy, and management must be determined according to the risk to the mother and fetus. In some cases, if renal function is seriously impaired before pregnancy, termination must be considered, particularly if hypertension is present. In the series discussed by Steel *et al* (1989), a good outcome was achieved in ongoing pregnancies when the creatinine clearance measured in a 24-hour urine sample was more than 40 ml/min in the first trimester. Renal function must be closely monitored throughout the pregnancy as deterioration may occur, necessitating the interruption of the pregnancy. In Oxford, all diabetic women complete 24-hour urine collections from the 24th week of pregnancy until delivery and one collection on returning for the 6-week postnatal visit. Distinguishing diabetic nephropathy from pre-eclampsia is difficult. Fetal growth retardation can occur with diabetic nephropathy as a result of the impaired ability of the uteroplacental blood vessels to accommodate the increasing blood flow required by the growing fetus.

☐ *Autonomic neuropathy*

Autonomic neuropathy can be demonstrated in diabetic women in pregnancy, but it is an uncommon clinical problem. Visceral neuropathy results from autonomic dysfunction of the stomach, bowel or bladder. Autonomic neuropathy may also affect vascular tone and cardiac rate. Gastroparesis can occasionally present with symptoms such as severe and continuing vomiting, leading to metabolic disturbance. The diagnosis is difficult as it is similar in appearance to morning sickness and hyperemesis gravidarum. This autonomic neuropathy can be associated with fetal loss (Macleod *et al* 1990).

☐ **Pregnancy complications**

Previously, the incidence of complications such as pre-eclampsia, antepartum haemorrhage and urinary tract infection was thought to be increased in a diabetic pregnancy. However, there is little evidence that this is the case (Cousins 1987). In the British Survey of Diabetic Pregnancies (Beard & Lowy 1982), the incidence of pre-eclampsia, 12 per cent among the established diabetic mothers, was the same for those mothers with gestational diabetes. The incidence for non-diabetic mothers is 1:10 of primigravidae and 1:100 of multigravidae (Cheston 1996). However, there was an increased risk to the fetus from any one of these three complications in association with diabetes. Pre-eclampsia and pyelonephritis have a prominent place in Pedersen's classification of prognostically bad signs for pregnancy in women with diabetes (Pedersen *et al* 1965).

☐ *Preterm labour*

Preterm (less than 37 weeks gestation) labour carries a reported threefold increased incidence in diabetic pregnancies (Molsted-Pedersen 1979). In the British Survey of Diabetic Pregnancies (Beard & Lowy 1982), half of the women with established diabetes were delivered before 38 weeks of gestation. In approximately two-thirds of the women, labour was induced or caesarean section performed, because of either fetal compromise or established practice. The remaining one third went into spontaneous labour for reasons likely to have been associated with polyhydramnios. The implications for the neonate are likely to be serious as a result of complications such as respiratory distress.

Preventing preterm labour with tocolytic drugs to suppress uterine contractions, and administering steroid therapy to aid lung maturation, can be contraindicated in diabetic pregnancies as a consequence of the resulting maternal metabolic disturbance, leading to ketoacidosis and insulin antagonism. Individual case reports have suggested that these therapies can be used safely provided that blood glucose levels are well controlled with intravenous insulin (Borberg *et al* 1978). This form of treatment is, however, only suitable for a short period, usually 24 hours, while the steroids are taking effect. It is felt that there is little advantage in delaying delivery as the treatment is potentially dangerous to the mother and fetus, especially if hyperglycaemia occurs (Maresh & Beard 1995).

☐ *Hypoglycaemia*

It has long been recognised that the first trimester is a period of glycaemic instability: insulin requirements may actually decrease, and hypoglycaemic episodes may become more frequent and more severe. The reason for this is thought to be alterations in substrate availability for maternal gluconeogenesis: early in non-diabetic pregnancies, a limited supply of amino acids has been shown to cause fasting hypoglycaemia (Felig & Lynch 1970). It is important at this stage for a family member to be taught how to inject glucagon should the woman become hypoglycaemic and be unable to swallow voluntarily. It is important to remember how distressing a severe hypoglycaemic attack can be for a pregnant woman and her family. Information on whom to contact and how to deal with this emergency situation is invaluable. It is very difficult at this stage of gestation to balance the need for tight glucose control with the aim of preventing hypoglycaemia. Kitzmiller *et al* (1991) did not find any increased rate of malformation among diabetic women who had experienced multiple hypoglycaemic attacks during the period of organogenesis. The role of hypoglycaemia in relation to birth defects remains controversial at this time.

☐ *Hyperglycaemia*

Weeks 3–6 after conception are the most important teratogenic phase for the fetus, during which poor control (hyperglycaemia) can lead to congenital malformations (Mills *et al* 1979). Furthermore, poor first trimester glucose control is linked with spontaneous miscarriage (Mills *et al* 1988a). The Diabetes in Early Pregnancy Study, which was conducted in the USA in the 1980s, invited participants to register within 21 days of conception (Mills 1988b). They were required to carry out home glucose monitoring and keep a diary of their results. Their infants were prospectively examined for defects, and no relationship was found with episodes of hypoglycaemia. This would seem to suggest that hyperglycaemia is the main cause of fetal malformation and spontaneous miscarriage.

The worst complication or endpoint of hyperglycaemia is diabetic ketoacidosis. Diabetic ketoacidosis is a real danger and may threaten the mother's life. This situation was described by Freinkel (1965) as accelerated starvation in pregnancy associated with heightened ketogenesis. Therefore pregnant women are at an increased risk of ketoacidosis, which causes substantial fetal and maternal mortality. In patients recovering from ketoacidosis, a marked reduction in red cell oxygen release is noted, which may account for the poor fetal prognosis (Maresh & Beard 1995). Primarily, ketoacidosis is caused by infection or an omitted insulin dose. It requires about 48 hours to develop in a well-controlled non-pregnant diabetic, but it may develop in 24 hours or less in a pregnant diabetic woman.

Fortunately, with home glucose monitoring and the ability to test the urine for ketones, this is a rare event. However, if the woman falls ill, ketonuria may be an early indication of problems. If this occurs, urgent medical aid and immediate transfer to hospital should be sought.

☐ Fetal complications

Currently, the rationale for the treatment of diabetes in pregnancy is concentrated on the prevention of three major complications: anomalies, stillbirth and macrosomia. All of these have been proved in the past to be glucose-related complications.

☐ *Spontaneous miscarriage*

Miodovnik *et al* suggested in 1984 that an increased incidence of miscarriage among women known to have diabetes before pregnancy was possibly related to poor diabetic control during embryogenesis, as determined by glycosylated haemoglobin measurement at 8–9 weeks. In contrast, no difference in the rate of miscarriage was found in a large prospective American study of diabetic women compared with control women seen by 21 days post-conception (Mills *et al* 1988b). However, those diabetic women who miscarried had higher fasting and postprandial glucose concentrations and glycosylated haemoglobin levels than did those with continuing pregnancies. Women who attend for pre-pregnancy counselling have also been shown to have no increase in miscarriage rate (Dicker *et al* 1988a). Poorly controlled diabetes thus does appear to be asssociated with an increased risk of miscarriage.

☐ *Congenital malformations*

There is an increased incidence of congenital malformation among the offspring of mothers with established diabetes, reported as varying from 2.7 per cent (Damm & Molsted-Pedersen 1989) to 11.9 per cent (Schneider *et al* 1980). The results from the British Survey of Diabetic Pregnancy (Beard & Lowy 1982) showed an incidence of 5.7 per cent among 664 mothers with established diabetes. The consensus is that there is about a threefold increase over the rate for the non-diabetic woman. Both minor and major malformations are more prevalent. Specific abnormalities are cardiac and neural tube defects, and the caudal regression syndrome (absence or hypoplasia of caudal structures), the latter being very rare (Kucera 1971). Various studies have reported an association between malformation and maternal hyperglycaemia. In 1964 Molsted-Pedersen *et al* showed an association between malformation rate and poor diabetic control. These and other findings suggest that there may be a critical concentration of blood glucose above which fetal malformations are more likely to develop. However, the relationship is not that simple since there is a considerable overlap between the glucose control and glycosylated haemoglobin values of women bearing abnormal babies and those with unaffected babies. Women with gestational diabetes do not have an increased incidence of malformation in their offspring, presumably because the metabolic disturbance of diabetes does not occur in the mother until later in pregnancy when organogenesis is complete (Malins 1979).

☐ Unexplained fetal death in utero

Despite improvements in diabetic care, unexplained fetal deaths in utero still accounted for 51 per cent of the perinatal mortality in the 1979–80 British Survey of mothers with diabetes (Lowy *et al* 1986). The aetiology is almost certainly multifactorial, but hyperglycaemia is likely to be important. Data obtained by direct fetal blood sampling using cordocentesis has provided more insight. Previously, studies on cord blood at delivery reported increased erythropoietin and haemoglobin concentrations and suggested a relationship with maternal glucose control (hyperglycaemia). This has been confirmed by cordocentesis, which has demonstrated that fetal thrombocytopenia occurs (Salvesen *et al* 1993).

Placental causes
Placental blood supply studies have suggested a decrease in flow of between 35 and 40 per cent in maternal diabetes (Nylund *et al* 1982). Initial umbilical cord Doppler flow measurements produced data that were difficult to interpret, but more recent studies indicate that values are within the normal range unless growth retardation or pre-eclampsia is present (Johnstone *et al* 1992). Placental abnormalities were reviewed in 1989 by Fox, who concluded that placental changes were not specific to diabetes and did not relate to the severity of the diabetes or its control. Placental oxygen transfer was reviewed by Madsen in 1986. Although there was an increase in maternal red blood cell content throughout all trimesters in diabetic pregnancy, an increasing concentration of maternal glycosylated haemoglobin was found to be associated with a small but signficant decrease in arterial oxygen saturation.

Therefore the conclusion is that no primary placental pathology occurs to cause fetal death in utero. It only appears to be implicated in growth retardation where there is superimposed pre-eclampsia.

Metabolic causes
Fetal acidosis has been implicated in fetal death. In work with sheep fetuses, it was reported that hyperglycaemia was of no significance to a well-oxygenated fetus, but with mild hypoxia there was a rapid fall in the pH with hyperglycaemia. As there is a correlation between fetal pH and arterial oxygen tension, one can suggest that sudden rises in maternal glucose could be enough to

cause fetal acidaemia and mild hypoxaemia, which might be sufficient to cause an irreversible pH decline and fetal demise (Shelley *et al* 1975).

The organomegaly induced by hyperinsulinaemia in the fetus of the diabetic mother will result in an increased oxygen demand, as has been shown in animal experiments (Carson *et al* 1980; Susa & Schwartz 1985).

Despite these current theories, the main cause for unexpected fetal death in utero remains unclear.

Thrombosis

In fetal haematology, there is both polycythaemia and thrombocytopenia, the latter probably resulting from platelet aggregation. The fetus is likely to be at increased risk of thrombotic episodes, which has been documented in post-mortem studies (Oppenheimer & Esterly 1965).

In conclusion, a number of factors are likely to be relevant in the consideration of an intrauterine death, the common link being poor diabetic control.

☐ Macrosomia

Studies have shown that tight glucose control can reduce the incidence of congenital abnormalities and stillbirth, but the incidence of macrosomia remains unchanged, varying between 20 and 50 per cent in most reported studies up to the 1980s (Gyves *et al* 1980). This issue has created the normoglycaemia paradox: the elimination of fetal mortality but no change in the incidence of macrosomia. The improvement in perinatal mortality rates is due to the improved approach to fetal lung maturation, increased antenatal surveillance and increased technology in neonatal units.

The clinical importance of fetal macrosomia, which is often associated with polyhydramnios, is that it may indicate poor diabetic control and an increased risk of perinatal mortality and morbidity. While most common in the insulin-dependent woman, it is also present in gestational diabetes. In addition, excessive fetal growth increases the risk of maternal and fetal trauma during vaginal delivery, particularly from shoulder dystocia. This is an exceedingly dangerous complication because of the rapid onset of fetal hypoxia (Coates 1995). If there is established macrosomia, caesarean section may be advised in order to reduce the degree of trauma.

Typically, between 25 and 40 per cent of infants of mothers with established diabetes have birthweights over the 90th percentile (Maresh, unpublished observations from 1985–86 at St Mary's Hospital, Manchester, UK). Excessive fetal growth rarely becomes obvious before 28 weeks gestation. The macrosomic baby of the diabetic mother is characteristically fat and plethoric, all organs, with the exception of the brain, being enlarged owing to an increase in cytoplasmic mass. Pederson's hypothesis (1977) is that the birthweight is increased through fetal pancreatic hyperplasia and hyperinsulinism. In the human fetus, subcutaneous fat content is markedly increased, the amount being directly related to the maternal plasma glucose concentration in the third trimester of pregnancy (Whitelaw 1977) and to glycosylated haemoglobin levels (Stubbs *et al* 1981). Morphological studies of the fetus of the diabetic mother have shown that the greater the percentage area of total pancreatic tissue occupied by insulin-secreting islet cells, the bigger the baby (Cardell 1953).

With the advent of ultrasound scanning in pregnancy and the use of cardiotocography, the ability to assess the state of fetal wellbeing in utero has been particularly important in the care of the fetus of the diabetic woman. Accurate assessment of fetal size has alerted the obstetrician to potentially 'at-risk' fetuses allowing for increased fetal surveillance. The biophysical profile (scoring for the presence of fetal movement, fetal tone, fetal breathing and liquor volume, and the resting cardiotocograph) has revolutionised the late pregnancy management of the diabetic woman and has more or less obviated the need for admission in late pregnancy (Dicker *et al* 1988b).

☐ Neonatal complications

☐ Respiratory dysfunction

Respiratory distress syndrome (RDS) of the newborn is a known complication of maternal diabetes. Bourbon and Farrell (1985) have suggested that fetal hyperinsulinism reduces pulmonary phospholipid production, leading to a deficiency of surfactant. RDS is becoming less common as a result of fewer preterm elective deliveries and better glucose control. It is being replaced by transient tachypnoea of the newborn, which is thought to result from delayed removal of fetal lung liquid and is quite commonly seen, especially following delivery by caesarean section. This is characterised by a rapid respiratory rate and transient cyanosis, usually disappearing within 24–36 hours of birth (Maresh & Beard 1995). The use of steroid therapy in women with diabetes is complicated. Their diabetic control is severely affected and they may require intravenous administration of insulin and glucose to reassert it. However, in certain situations, steroid therapy may be required, and this may cause the decreased rate of respiratory distress seen.

☐ Hypoglycaemia

Hypoglycaemia is usually asymptomatic in the newborn baby. Plasma glucose concentrations of less than 2 mmol/l without evidence of systemic disturbances are common. The condition is caused by endogenous hyperinsulinism developing during fetal life that only becomes evident when the fetus is deprived of its maternal supply of glucose. Symptomatic hypoglycaemia increases the baby's likelihood of cerebral damage. This is preceded by jitteriness and convulsions, or simply by limpness or an abnormal cry (Gentz *et al* 1969). By encouraging early feeding and performing regular glucose recordings in the newborn, the condition can be detected and treated before symptoms develop. A plasma glucose value of less than 1 mmol/l in the newborn is an indication for the intravenous administration of glucose to lower the risk of brain damage.

☐ *Polycythaemia and jaundice*

Polycythaemia is more common in the infants of diabetic mothers. A venous haematocrit of greater than 65 per cent is considered abnormal. Salvesen *et al* (1993) have demonstrated fetal polycythaemia related to poor maternal diabetic control through studies using cordocentesis. The clinical consequence of polycythaemia is an increased blood viscosity leading to increased cardiac work and microcirculatory disturbances (Maresh & Beard 1995). The hyperviscosity within the pulmonary bed may be a factor contributing to respiratory distress in the newborn and might also explain the increased incidence of renal vein thrombosis and necrotising enterocolitis. The destruction of many erythrocytes and the relative immaturity of the liver enzyme systems, which concentrate the bilirubin, predispose these babies to a higher incidence of jaundice. The rate of jaundice varies, but typically 19 per cent would have bilirubin values exceeding 15 mg/dl (Kitzmiller *et al* 1978). These conclusions led Persson *et al* (1978) to recommend early clamping of the umbilical cord and exchange transfusion if the haematocrit exceeded 70 per cent.

The recommendations made by the Pregnancy and Neonatal Care Group (Jardine Brown *et al* 1996) were that a paediatrician should be present at the delivery of all diabetic women. The infant does not routinely need to be admitted to the special care nursery unless a neonatal problem is apparent or anticipated. It is recommended that the baby should remain with the mother to facilitate bonding and early breastfeeding. Routine neonatal blood glucose monitoring should be performed for the first 24 hours following delivery to detect hypoglycaemia. Finally, it is suggested that, if symptoms of RDS develop, surfactant should be administered early.

■ Gestational diabetes

Some pregnant women have certain features in their family, medical or obstetric backgrounds that may predispose them to developing diabetes in pregnancy. The following are all risk factors:

- A family history of diabetes;

- Maternal obesity (>120 per cent ideal body weight);

- A previous large baby (>4 kg);

- A previous unexplained stillbirth;

- A previous abnormal glucose tolerance (Maresh & Beard 1995);

- Gestational diabetes in a previous pregnancy (Oats *et al* 1988);

- Evidence of macrosomia in the current pregnancy;

- Polyhydramnios;

- Maternal age >35 years (McFarland & Case 1985);

- Pregnancy-induced hypertension.

Some of these factors can be established at a booking visit by the midwife, alerting her to the possibility of potential gestational diabetes.

☐ Physiology and pathophysiology

Pregnancy induces profound metabolic alterations in every woman, whether or not she has diabetes, which tend to become more pronounced with advancing gestational age. It seems likely that these changes are adaptive, ensuring the optimal environment for fetal growth and development. Normally, maternal glucose homeostasis is maintained over a 24-hour period. In both early and late pregnancy, the glucose concentration stays constant, at between 4.0 and 6.0 mmol/l, except after meals. This degree of homeostasis is only maintained by doubling the secretion of insulin from the end of the first to the third trimester of pregnancy (Gillmer *et al* 1975). Although there is some disagreement on whether glucose tolerance normally decreases as pregnancy advances, longitudinal studies have shown glucose concentrations to be increased postprandially and decreased with fasting in pregnancy.

☐ Definition of gestational diabetes mellitus

The current widely accepted definition of gestational diabetes agreed at the Second International Workshop Conference on Gestational Diabetes Mellitus (1985) is 'carbohydrate intolerance of variable severity with onset or first recognition during the present pregnancy'. This rather vague definition was coupled with the glucose tolerance criteria for the diagnosis of gestational diabetes established by O'Sullivan and Mahan (1964), using an 100 g oral glucose load.

During the Pregnancy and Neonatal Care Group's study into diabetes in the UK (Jardine Brown *et al* 1996), the confusion over how to define and diagnose gestational diabetes became apparent. Only 32.8 per cent of units were using routine blood glucose testing for antenatal screening and, of these, only 5.8 per cent were using the 50 g oral glucose challenge test (GCT) advocated in the USA. In contrast, 25.9 per cent of all units were using random blood glucose testing, mainly at the booking visit or between 28 and 32 weeks gestation. These data indicate that antenatal blood glucose testing is used in a minority of obstetric units in this country, and that the 50 g GCT has not been favoured by British obstetricians.

Routine urine testing for glycosuria was, however, performed antenatally in 89.4 per cent of units. This was followed by one or more of the following blood glucose tests: a 75 g oral glucose tolerance test (GTT), a random blood glucose level, fasting blood glucose level, 50 g oral GCT, and pre- and or post-meal glucose measurements.

The Pregnancy and Neonatal Care Group recommended a screening protocol for gestational diabetes:

1. Urine should be tested for glycosuria at every antenatal visit.

2. Timed random laboratory blood glucose measurements (fasting, 2 hours postprandially, or more than 2 hours postprandially) should be made:
   - Whenever glycosuria (1+ or more) is detected;
   - At the booking visit;
   - At 28 weeks gestation.

3. A 75 g oral GTT with laboratory venous blood glucose measurements should be performed if the timed random blood glucose concentrations are:
   - >6 mmol/l in the fasting state or 2 hours after food; *or*
   - >7 mmol/l within 2 hours of taking food.

4. Interpretation of the 75g oral GTT during pregnancy should be made:

	Plasma glucose*	
	Fasting	2-hour
Diabetes	>8 mmol/l	>11 mmol/l
Gestational	6–8 mmol/l	9–11 mmol/l
Normal	<6 mmol/l	<9 mmol/l

* Upper limits of normal above which interventions should occur.

These measurements should ideally be made after 75 g of 'Lucozade' or its equivalent and must be made in a laboratory. The results provide evidence of insulin-dependent diabetes or gestational diabetes and confirm the normal levels. (Jardine Brown *et al* 1996).

Women with an abnormal 75 g oral GTT will usually require insulin treatment and should ideally be taught to use a home blood glucose meter to maintain their blood glucose below 6 mmol/l in the preprandial state.

Lawson and Rajaram (1994) considered the psychosocial conse-quences of gestational diabetes, exploring the meaning that women attached to the disorder. They found that gestational diabetes had a profound effect on the respondents' imagery of diabetes as a debilitating disease associated with blindness, amputations and premature death. There was an increased anxiety throughout the pregnancy and at the 6-week postnatal examination. This needs to be considered when caring for women with gestational diabetes.

■ Recommendations for clinical practice in the light of currently available evidence

These are based on the main findings and suggestions made by the Preg-nancy and Neonatal Care Group for the St Vincent Declaration (Jardine Brown *et al* 1996).

1. Dietary recommendations

All diabetic women should be offered pre-pregnancy dietetic advice. Diets with high levels of complex carbohydrate and soluble fibre and reduced levels of saturated fat have been shown to enhance insulin sensitivity and lower postprandial blood glucose concentrations. The benefits of soluble fibre are most apparent when it is taken in conjunction with at least 50 per cent energy from carbohydrate. Levels of dietary fibre of 30–50 g per day are recommended, but, if this proves difficult to achieve, an increase in monosat-urated fat intake is preferable to one of simple carbohydrate or saturated fat. An energy prescription of 30–35 kcal/kg pre-pregnant ideal body weight is recommended, although this should be flexible since women may alter their activities during pregnancy and gain or lose weight in the first trimester.

The recommendation for all women planning a pregnancy is to take a folate supplement of 0.4 mg each day for at least a month before concep-tion to reduce the risk of neural tube defects. This advice is especially relevant for diabetic women because of the increased risk of neural tube defects in their babies.

Open access to dietetic counselling should be available in all diabetic antenatal clinics.

2. The roles of the diabetes specialist midwife and nurse

All centres caring for pregnant diabetic women should provide a diabetes specialist midwife and nurse who should be available to provide support and advice both in the clinic and by telephone. The specialist nurse in the diabetic clinic should identify those women likely to become pregnant and encourage adequate contraception until optimal diabetic control has been achieved. The specialist midwife and nurse should help to educate the woman to achieve optimal diabetic control during pregnancy and should act as a link between the woman and all those involved in her care, ensuring that the lead professional responsible for her care is identified at each stage in the pregnancy. The specialist midwife and nurse should be engaged in the practical training of other professionals in the care of the pregnant diabetic woman.

3. Achieving diabetic control

Opinions on the standard of glycaemic control that is necessary in pregnancy vary, but most studies reveal that the upper limit of normal for fasting venous plasma glucose in the third trimester of pregnancy is between 5.5 and 6.0 mmol/l; this latter figure therefore appears to be a reasonable goal for women with insulin-dependent diabetes. There is a need in the medical management of the pregnancies of women with diabetes to achieve optimal glycaemic control. This can, however, only be achieved within a well-organised clinical service in which the woman is provided with a blood glucose meter and test strips to perform home blood glucose monitoring six times a day twice a week, or more often if required.

The report of the Pregnancy and Neonatal Care Group (Jardine Brown *et al* 1996) identified a need to encourage subspecialisation by obsteticians to improve standards of care, especially in the smaller maternity units. Special clinics should be held at which all members of the team caring for diabetic women should be present. This would enhance the standards of care, not least by improving convenience for the woman.

4. Antenatal obstetric surveillance

The report (Jardine Brown *et al* 1996) identified a number of problems with antenatal and intrapartum care. There was an underutilisation of ultrasound to assess the fetal biophysical profile (and hence wellbeing) in late pregnancy. The timing of delivery in some units was unnecessarily early, while in others it was needlessly prolonged, with possible risk to the fetus. In some maternity units, diabetic women were receiving inadequate carbohydrate during labour, while in others there was a risk of fluid overload and water intoxication owing to the administration of excessive amounts of hypotonic dextrose solution. There was a need for revised protocols for infusions during labour. Continuous fetal heart rate monitoring and fetal blood samples should be available during labour for all diabetic women. Spontaneous vaginal delivery should be encouraged wherever possible for diabetic women.

5. Postnatal care and contraception

Prophylactic antibiotics should be given to diabetic women after caesarean section because of the increased risk of wound infection. All diabetic women should be seen and offered appropriate contraceptive advice at the 6-week postnatal examination (Jardine Brown *et al* 1996).

6. The woman's perspective

A register of specialist antenatal clinics should be made available to diabetic women wishing to become pregnant. More information is required about diabetic pregnancy and its management. Jardine Brown *et al* (1996) suggest that more information should be available in diabetic centres, chemists and GP surgeries. In order to exercise more choice, the diabetic woman should have access to information about pregnancy management and outcome at the hospitals where she could have her baby.

■ Practice check

- Are you aware of the risk factors for gestational diabetes? Do you ensure that these factors are discussed while taking a booking history?

- Do you know the diabetic women covered by your GP's practice? Have they any access to preconceptual care, maybe through communication with the diabetic specialist nurses?

- Do you know how to obtain and administer glucagon? Could you teach a family member to be aware of the symptoms of hypoglycaemia and how to act appropriately?

- Are you aware of the many medical and obstetric risk factors faced by an insulin-dependent diabetic woman and how these can affect her pregnancy and fetus?

- Do you know how to use a home blood glucose monitoring meter and how to act appropriately on the results? Do you know whom to contact at the hospital or how to contact the diabetic clinic? What specialist facilities are available locally for the care of pregnant women with diabetes?

- Are you aware of the dangers of hyperglycaemia? Do you check for ketonuria in the diabetic women in your care?

- Are you aware of the worries and fears of women diagnosed with gestational diabetes during pregnancy? How can you help them come to terms with these worries? (Lawson & Rajaram 1994)

- Are you aware of how to obtain further information on the care of diabetics in pregnancy and how to keep your practice up to date?

☐ Acknowledgements

My thanks to Miss Geraldine Gaffney for her help in compiling this chapter and indicating where to find the information. Thanks also to Mr MDG Gillmer for all the support and assistance he has given in my increasing awareness of the implications for midwives caring for diabetics, and to the diabetic women, who always amaze me!

■ References

Beard RW, Lowy C 1982 The British Survey of Diabetic Pregnancies. British Journal of Obstetrics and Gynaecology   89: 783–6 (Commentary)

Borberg C, Gillmer MDG, Beard RW, Oakley NW 1978 Metabolic effects of beta-sympathomimetic drugs and dexamethasone in normal and diabetic pregnancy. British Journal of Obstetrics and Gynaecology   85: 184–9

Bourbon JR, Farrell PM 1985 Fetal lung development in the diabetic pregnancy. Pediatric Research   19: 253–67

Cardell BA 1953 Hypertrophy and hyperplasia of the pancreatic islets in new born infants. Journal of Pathology and Bacteriology   66: 335–8

Carson BS, Phillips AF, Simmons MA 1980 Effects of a sustained insulin infusion upon glucose uptake and oxygenation of the ovine fetus. Pediatric Research   14: 147–52

Coates T 1995 Shoulder dystocia. In Alexander J, Levy V, Roch S (eds) Aspects of midwifery practice: a research-based approach. Macmillan, Basingstoke, Ch 4, pp69–93

Cousins L Pregnancy complications among diabetic women: review 1965–1985. Obstetrical and Gynecological Survey 1987   42: 140–9

Damm P, Molsted-Pedersen L, 1989 Significant decrease in congenital malformations in newborn infants of an unselected population of diabetic women. American Journal of Obstetrics and Gynecology   161: 1163–7

Dibble CM, Kochenour NK, Worley RJ, Tyler FH, Swartz M 1982 Effect of pregnancy on diabetic retinopathy. Obstetrics and Gynecology   59: 699–704

Dicker D, Feldberg D, Samuel N, Yeshaya A, Karp M, Goldman JA 1988a Spontaneous abortion in patients with insulin-dependent diabetes mellitus. The effect of preconceptional diabetic control. American Journal of Obstetrics and Gynecology   158: 1161–4

Dicker D, Feldberg D, Yeshaya A, Peleg D, Karp M, Goldman JA 1988b Fetal surveillance in insulin-dependent diabetic pregnancy: predictive value of the Biophysical Profile. American Journal of Obstetrics and Gynecology   159: 800–4

Drury PL, Doddridge M 1992 Pre-pregnancy clinics for diabetic women. Lancet 340: 919

Duncan MJ 1882 On puerperal diabetes. Transactions of the Obstetric Society of London   24: 256–85

Felig P, Lynch V 1970 Starvation in human pregnancy: hypoglycaemia, hypoinsulinaemia and hyperketonaemia. Science   170: 990–2

Forrester JV, Towler HMA, Pearson DWM 1989 Pregnancy and diabetic retinopathy. In Sutherland HW, Stowers JM, Pearson DWM (eds) Carbohydrate metabolism in pregnancy and the newborn, vol. IV. Springer-Verlag, Berlin, pp189–200

Fox H 1989 The placenta in diabetes mellitus. In Sutherland HW, Stowes JM, Pearson DWM (eds) Carbohydrate metabolism in pregnancy and the newborn, vol IV. Springer-Verlag, Berlin, pp109–17

Freinkel N 1965 Effects of the conceptus on maternal metabolism in pregnancy. In Leibel BS, Wrenshall GA (eds) On the nature and treatment of diabetes. Excerpta Medica Foundation, Amsterdam, pp679–91

Fuhrmann K, Reiher H, Semmler K, Fischer F, Fischer M, Glockner E 1983 Prevention of congenital malformations in infants of insulin dependent diabetic mothers. Diabetes Care   6: 219–23

Gentz J, Persson B, Zetterstrom R 1969 On the diagnosis of symptomatic neonatal hypoglycaemia. Acta Paediatrica Scandinavica   58: 449–59

Gillmer MDG, Beard RW, Brooke FM, Oakley NW 1975 Carbohydrate metabolism in pregnancy, part II, Relation between maternal glucose tolerance and glucose metabolism in the newborn. British Medical Journal   iii: 402–4

Gyves MT, Schulman PK, Merkatz IR 1980 Results of individualized intervention in gestational diabetes. Diabetes Care   3: 495–6

Jardine Brown C, Dawson A, Dodds R *et al* 1996: Report of the Pregnancy and Neonatal Care Group. Diabetic Medicine   13: s43–s53

Johnstone FD, Steel JM, Haddad NG, Hoskins PR, Greer IA, Chambers S 1992 Doppler umbilical artery flow velocity waveforms in diabetic pregnancy. British Journal of Obstetrics and Gynaecology   99: 135–40

Kitzmiller JL, Gavin LA, Gin GD 1991 Preconception management of diabetes continued through early pregnancy prevents the excess frequency of major congenital anomalies in infants of diabetic mothers. Journal of the American Medical Association   265: 731

Kitzmiller JL, Cloherty JP, Younger MD *et al* 1978 Diabetic pregnancy and perinatal morbidity. American Journal of Obstetrics and Gynecology   131: 560–80

Kucera J 1971 Rate and type of congenital anomalies among offspring in diabetic women. Journal of Reproductive Medicine 7: 61–70

Lawson EJ, Rajaram S 1994 A transformed pregnancy: the psychosocial consequences of gestational diabetes. Sociology of Health and Illness   16(4): 536–62

Lowy C, Beard RW, Goldschmidt J 1986 Congenital malformations in babies of diabetic mothers. Diabetic Medicine   3: 458–62

McFarland KF, Case CA 1985 The relationship of maternal age to gestational diabetes. Diabetes Care   8: 598–600

Macleod AF, Smith SA, Sonksen PH, Lowy C 1990 The problem of autonomic neuropathy in diabetic pregnancy. Diabetic Medicine   7: 80–2

Madsen H 1986 Fetal oxygenation in diabetic pregnancy. Danish Medical Bulletin 33: 64–74

Malins J 1979 Fetal anomalies related to carbohydrate metabolism. The epidemiological approach. In Sutherland HW, Stowers JM (eds) Carbohydrate metabolism in pregnancy and the newborn. Springer-Verlag, Berlin, pp229–46

Maresh M, Beard RW 1995 Medical disorders in obstetric practice, 3rd edn. Blackwell, Oxford, p423

Mills JL, Baker L, Goldman AS 1979 Malformations in infants of diabetic mothers occur before the seventh gestational week. Diabetes   28: 292–3

Mills JL, Knopp RH, Simpson JL et al 1988a Lack of relation of increased malformation rates in infants of diabetic mothers to glycaemic control during organogenesis. New England Journal of Medicine 318: 671–6

Mills JL, Simpson JL, Driscoll SG et al 1988b Incidence of spontaneous abortion among normal women and insulin-dependent diabetic women whose pregnancies were identified within 21 days of conception. New England Journal of Medicine 319: 1617–23

Miodovnik M, Lavin JP, Knowles HC, Holroyde J, Stys SJ 1984 Spontaneous abortion among insulin-dependent diabetic women. American Journal of Obstetrics and Gynecology 150: 372–6

Molsted-Pedersen L 1979 Preterm labour and perinatal mortality in diabetic pregnancy. Obstetric considerations. In Sutherland HW, Stowers JM (eds) Carbohydrate metabolism in pregnancy and the newborn. Springer-Verlag, Berlin, pp392–406

Molsted-Pedersen L, Tygstrup I, Pedersen J 1964 Congenital malformations in newborn infants of diabetic women. Correlation with maternal diabetic vascular complications. Lancet i: 1124–6

Nylund L, Lunell NO, Lewander R, Persson B, Sarby B, Thornström S 1982 Uteroplacental blood flow in diabetic pregnancy: measurements with indium 113m and a computer-linked gamma camera. American Journal of Obstetrics and Gynecology 144: 298–302

Oats JN, Beischer NA, Grant PT 1988 The emergence of diabetes and impaired glucose tolerance in women who had gestational diabetes. In Weiss PAM, Coustan DR (eds) Gestational diabetes. Springer, Vienna, pp199–207

Oppenheimer EH, Esterly JR 1965 Thrombosis in the newborn: comparison between diabetic and non-diabetic mothers. Journal of Pediatrics 67: 549

O'Sullivan JB, Mahan CM 1964 Criteria for the oral glucose tolerance test in pregnancy. Diabetes 13: 278–85

Pedersen J 1977 The pregnant diabetic and her newborn: problems and management. Munksgaard, Copenhagen

Pedersen J, Molsted-Pedersen L 1965 Prognosis of the outcome of pregnancies in diabetics. A new classification. Acta Endocrinologica 50: 70–4

Persson B, Gentz J, Lunell NO 1978 Diabetes in pregnancy. In Scarpelli EM, Cosmi EV (eds) Reviews in perinatal medicine 2: 1–55

Salvesen DR, Brudenell JM, Proudler AJ, Crook D, Nicolaides KH 1993 Fetal pancreatic Beta-cell function in pregnancies complicated by maternal diabetes mellitus: relationship to fetal acidaemia and macrosomia. American Journal of Obstetrics and Gynecology 168: 88–94

Schneider JM, Curet LB, Olson RW, Stay G 1980 Ambulatory care of the pregnant diabetic. Obstetrics and Gynecology 56:144–9

Second International Workshop Conference on Gestational Diabetes Mellitus 1985 Summary and recommendations. Diabetes 34(supplement 2): 123–6

Shelley HJ, Bassett JM, Miller RDG 1975 Control of carbohydrate metabolism in the fetus and newborn. British Medical Bulletin 31: 37–43

Steel JM, Johnstone FD, Smith AF 1989 Prepregnancy preparation. In Sutherland HW, Stowers JM, Pearson DWM (eds) Carbohydrate metabolism in pregnancy and the newborn, vol. IV. Springer-Verlag, Berlin, pp129-39

Steel JM, Johnstone FD, Smith AF 1990 Can prepregnancy care of diabetic women reduce the risk of abnormal babies? British Medical Journal 301: 1070–4

Stubbs SM, Leslie RDG, John PN 1981 Fetal macrosomia and maternal diabetic control in pregnancy. British Medical Journal 282: 439–40

Susa JB, Schwartz R 1985 Effects of hyperinsulinaemia in the primate fetus. Diabetes 34(supplement 2): 36–41

Whitelaw A 1977 Subcutaneous fat in newborn infants of diabetic mothers: an indication of quality of diabetic control. Lancet i: 15–18

■ Suggested further reading

Gillmer MDG 1996 Management of pre-existing disorders in pregnancy: diabetes mellitus. Prescribers' Journal   36(3): 159–64

Gillmer MDG, Bickerton NJ 1995 Advance in the management of diabetes in pregnancy: success through simplicity. In Bonnar J (ed.) Recent advances in obstetrics and gynaecology. Churchill Livingstone, Edinburgh, pp51–78

Kuhl C 1991 Aetiology of gestational diabetes. In Oats JN (ed.) Diabetes in pregnancy. Baillière's Clinical Obstetrics and Gynaecology, 20(3): 279–92

Landon MB 1993 Clinics in Perinatology. Diabetes in Pregnancy   20(3)

Oats JN 1991 Diabetes in pregnancy. Baillière's Clinical Obstetrics and Gynaecology 5(2)

Chapter 7

Care during the second stage of labour

Rona McCandlish

Entering the second stage of labour can be an almost overwhelming experience for a labouring woman. Some find it liberating and exciting – at last the end of labour is coming, they can push, something is happening; for others, it is the hardest part of labour, when they can become demoralised, feeling they can't go on, even believing they are going to die (Halldorsdóttir & Karlsdóttir 1996).

For a midwife, being with a woman through this phase means staying with her, sharing in the mounting excitement and tension as the birth comes closer. The positive effects of having someone empathetic and supportive with a labouring woman are well documented (Hodnett 1995), but such a companion does not necessarily have to be a midwife. The skill of the midwife at this stage in labour involves offering appropriate professional care. What this actually constitutes will be influenced by a variety of factors, including the individual woman's own wishes, the experience of her attending midwife, the location in which she is labouring and local practice guidelines.

The purpose of this chapter is to highlight research-based information about some key aspects of care. Midwives are increasingly active in challenging their own established practices, and therefore much of the evidence discussed comes from midwifery-led studies. Aspects of care examined include the onset and duration of the second stage, 'pushing' policies, maternal position and perineal management.

■ **It is assumed that you are already aware of the following:**

- The anatomy of the pelvic floor and related structures;

- The physiological changes accompanying the second stage of labour;

- The terms midline and medio-lateral episiotomy.

■ The onset of the second stage of labour

The second stage of labour begins when the cervix reaches full dilatation and ends when the baby's body is completely born. The rate and intensity of contractions may alter so that, for some women, they may be more frequent and intense than they were during the first stage, while for others they come less often with a lengthy gap between.

At the onset of the second stage, a woman may express an overwhelming urge to bear down. This impulse is not, of itself, a certain indication that the woman has reached the end of the first stage of labour. Up to two-thirds of women may experience an expulsive urge before they reach full cervical dilatation (Roberts *et al* 1987), and it may be possible to help these women to resist this urge by staying by their sides and talking them through each contraction. Some practitioners believe that assisting the woman to change position will also help; for example, if she is in an upright position, adopting a lateral posture or moving to an all fours position may reduce the urgency to push (Kitzinger 1991).

■ Duration of the second stage of labour

The fundamental requirement of midwifery is that the midwife should provide care for a mother and baby during the antenatal, intranatal and postnatal periods, and that she should be able to recognise and seek appropriate help when there is deviation from the norm (UKCC 1993). Recording the onset and monitoring the duration of the second stage of labour are important components of the observations that enable a midwife to assess whether or not labour is progressing normally.

A number of retrospective studies have attempted to determine an upper 'limit' for the length of normal second stage in order to define when active intervention should be considered (Friedman 1955, 1956; Saunders *et al* 1992; Meticoglou *et al* 1995; Albers *et al* 1996a). Friedman's influential survey carried out in the early 1950s established a mean length of second stage for primiparous and multiparous women respectively of 0.95 hours (upper 'limit' 2.5 hours) and 0.29 hours (upper 'limit' 0.83 hours). However, the sample he used included women who could not have been expected to have normal labours, for example women with twin pregnancies and some who had breech presentations. Despite this, these data have been widely used to guide policies for clinical care in normal labour. A national survey carried out in England (Garcia & Garforth 1989) identified that the upper 'limits' of 1 hour for nulliparous women and half an hour for multiparous women were in general use.

Recent retrospective studies have questioned the validity of Friedman's conclusions (Albers *et al* 1996a) and have suggested that it would be appropriate to revise upwards the expected duration of the second stage. Meticoglou *et al* (1995) propose that an upper limit for the second stage should not be determined simply on the length of time since full dilatation but must also take into account signs of progress and the condition of the mother and baby. In their retrospective study of routinely collected maternity data in a Canadian hospital, only 10–15 per cent of the small number of women who experienced 5 hours in the second stage gave birth spontaneously. They conclude that, in the absence of clear signs of progress, there is no justification for continuing conservative management beyond this upper time limit, and therefore active intervention should be undertaken for the overwhelming majority of women who have spent 5 hours in the second stage.

There will be few occasions when a midwife will attend a woman whose second stage lasts as long as 5 hours, and it is easy to become side-tracked trying to establish an upper limit that is irrelevant for the overwhelming majority of childbearing women. The evidence does suggest that there may be conservative limits in place in many maternity units (Garcia & Garforth 1989), so the challenge is to think beyond such simplistic boundaries and instead use observations about the duration of the second stage in the context of other assessments about the progress of an individual woman's labour as the basis for decisions about labour management.

Arbitrarily limiting the length of this stage of labour for all women is likely to subject some to inappropriate interventions and therefore cause more harm than good. If labour is progressing and there are no signs of maternal or fetal problems, the observation that the second stage is 'long' is not, of itself, an indication for active intervention.

While the urge to define the safe upper 'limit' of the duration of the second stage continues to cause controversy, some women experience the opposite problem: a precipitate labour. This can be an extremely distressing and traumatising event for the woman and her partner. Precipitate labour involves strong contractions from the onset and progresses to delivery within an hour (Williams 1993). The care of women who experience precipitate delivery has not been subject to evaluation and therefore remains an area in which pragmatic practice and custom prevail. The principles of management are to remain with the woman to comfort and support her, and to try to control the birth of the baby's head as much as possible in order to minimise sudden expulsion, with its concomitant risks of cerebral trauma for the newborn and of perineal laceration for the mother.

■ Position for delivery

In the UK, the term 'alternative' birth position generally means one other than recumbent or semirecumbent and reflects the dominance of these positions among women who give birth in hospital (Garcia *et al* 1986). Women giving birth in other contexts and cultures may commonly use different positions (Dunham *et al* 1991; Gareberg *et al* 1994). The position adopted by a woman can be affected by a range of factors, for example her personal preference, the experience and confidence of her midwife, whether she has an effective epidural in operation and the level of her spine at which this is sited, and whether she is using immersion in water during the birth.

There is good evidence that adopting a dorsal position induces maternal aortocaval compression and consequent hypotension, which in turn compromises fetal oxygen levels (Kurtz *et al* 1982). These effects are likely to be potentiated by prolonged adoption of this position and by conventional epidural anaesthetic (Aldrich *et al* 1995a). Changing position to the left lateral may reduce these problems (Humphrey *et al* 1973; Aldrich *et al* 1995a). The evidence generated from these two observational studies and from two small randomised controlled trials (Humphrey *et al* 1973; Johnstone *et al* 1987) indicates that further research is required to establish whether or not there are significant differences between these positions in terms of neonatal or maternal outcome. However, Aldrich *et al* (1995b) concluded that the small, clinically insignificant decrease observed in fetal blood oxygenation in their study of 14 women in normal, uncomplicated labour might become more important if the fetus were already in a poor condition. The evidence so far suggests that a dorsal position may be associated with poorer fetal outcomes, but further research is required to confirm this.

Most studies that have compared different positions during the second stage among women not using epidural anaesthesia have used some kind of mechanical aid to enable the women allocated to an upright position to maintain this posture. These range from a specially designed cushion (Gardosi *et al* 1989) or chair (Stewart 1991) to wedges (Chan 1963) and pillows (McManus and Calder 1978).

A systematic review of the 17 randomised controlled trials that evaluated the effects of position during the second stage of labour (Nikodem 1995a) concluded that women who adopt an upright posture are likely to report less discomfort and intolerable pain, to experience a shorter second stage of labour (in the absence of oxytocic augmentation), to report that bearing down was less difficult and to have more chance of a spontaneous birth with fewer perineal or vaginal tears. However, there was an increased risk of labial tear, and studies in which birthing chairs were used to facilitate an upright position reported that women allocated to this were more likely to have an estimated blood loss of 500 ml or more (Stewart *et al* 1983; Turner *et al* 1986; Stewart & Spiby 1989; Waldenstrom & Gottvall 1991). Waldenstrom and Gottvall (1991), in common with the previous investigators, suggested that this finding could be explained by the imprecision of estimated blood loss for the group allocated to receive 'conventional care' compared with the possibility of more accurate measurement for the group allocated to a birthing chair. Midwives attending a woman using a birthing chair had the opportunity of collecting blood in a container held below the chair and therefore might have measured the amount lost more accurately. Waldenstrom and Gottvall (1991) also discussed the possibility that greater blood loss in the women allocated to upright posture could be explained by 'quicker emptying of blood from the uterus, and especially from the vagina'. Sleep *et al* (1989) suggested that the tendency to increased blood loss was more likely to be due to obstructed venous return to the perineal tissues associated with the upright position and its effect on bleeding from perineal trauma. In an attempt to establish a more objective measure of blood loss among women participating in a randomised controlled trial comparing the use of a birthing bed and a conventional bed, Crowley *et al* (1991) recorded haemoglobin levels for participants at 3–4 days after birth. However, this study did not show any significant difference in this outcome.

Some studies have asked women their views about the posture they adopted for birth (Gardosi *et al* 1989; Crowley *et al* 1991; Waldenstrom & Gottvall 1991). Most women who gave birth in a recumbent position said they would prefer to adopt a different position for a subsequent birth, while those allocated to an upright position would opt for that again.

It appears that there is no convincing evidence that use of an upright position of itself increases the risk of clinically important blood loss or any other serious maternal or neonatal morbidity. However, restricting the position a woman is able to adopt, so that she is unable to change position when she wishes, may be associated with such unwanted outcomes.

■ Pushing during the second stage of labour

In the absence of an effective epidural anaesthetic, it is reasonable for a woman to expect that she will experience active expulsive contractions towards the end of her labour. Until recently, it was established practice in many institutional settings for the attending midwife to give specific instructions about how the woman should breath during contractions. These instructions aim to direct and control expulsive contractions and 'organise' pushing. The midwife tells the woman to wait for the beginning of a contraction, take a deep breath, hold the breath and bear down for as long as possible, snatch another breath before the end of the contraction and bear down again. This series of actions, the Valsalva manoeuvre, is also characterised by 'forcible exhalation against the closed glottis' (Sweet 1992).

This 'organised pushing' is intended to maximise the woman's efforts and bring the labour to an end as efficiently as possible. However, breath-holding increases maternal intrathoracic pressure and initially raises and then lowers her blood pressure (Bassell *et al* 1980); consequently fetal oxygenation may be reduced (Knauth & Haloburdo 1986; Aldrich *et al* 1995b). These changes seem not to be important if the baby is healthy but may lead to morbidity if the fetus is already compromised or if maternal effort is prolonged.

The problems associated with organised pushing have stimulated a reconsideration of this aspect of care in favour of the midwife supporting and enabling rather than leading spontaneous maternal effort. Such support requires the midwife to understand what is likely to happen if she does not intervene, and to do this she needs to have information about the 'normal' pattern of expulsive effort.

In an observational study of 31 healthy nulliparous women, Roberts *et al* (1987) reported this pattern as being five to six pushes lasting between 4 and 6 seconds per contraction. Further information about spontaneous pushing was reported as part of a small pilot trial involving 32 women (Thomson 1993). Fifteen nulliparous women in normal labour were randomly allocated to spontaneous effort and compared with 17 women randomly allocated to directed pushing. The 15 women allocated to the spontaneous group were described as using a mixture of open and closed glottis pushing. These women did not always appear to have an expulsive urge with each contraction and the expulsive urge did not coincide with the beginning of, or cease before the end of, the contraction (Thomson 1995).

That study was designed to test research tools to be used in a larger trial and was therefore too small to detect true differences between the groups in terms of maternal or neonatal outcome. However, a similar randomised controlled trial involving 306 primiparous women in normal term labour was carried out in Denmark (Parnell *et al* 1993) and found no significant differences in the duration of second stage, fetal arterial pH (as assessed from an umbilical sample taken immediately after birth) or perineal trauma.

Organised pushing may be appropriately used to assist women who have an effective epidural anaesthetic during the second stage because they will not experience spontaneous expulsive contractions. The timing of directed pushing has been considered in a meta-analysis of the results of trials that have compared early (as soon as full dilatation has been diagnosed) and late (when the vertex is visible at the introitus) pushing among women with an epidural (Nikodem 1995b). No increase in fetal distress among women encouraged to bear down early was identified; however, operative delivery was more common in that group, with significantly more rotational forceps deliveries. The duration of the second stage was significantly shorter in the 'early' group, and there were no differences in rates of perineal trauma. On the basis of these findings, there appears to be no evidence to support the routine use of early bearing down among women who have an effective epidural anaesthetic during the second stage.

■ Prevention of perineal trauma

Some degree of perineal trauma is sustained by the majority of women who have a spontaneous birth, and many experience considerable discomfort and pain during the immediate postnatal period (Sleep *et al* 1984). These problems can affect mobility, inhibit normal bowel function and interfere with many activities, such as the ability to adopt a comfortable position in which to breastfeed. In the longer term, women may experience dyspareunia and other sexual difficulties (Sleep & Grant 1987; Glazener *et al* 1995).

A major focus for midwifery care during the second stage is management to try to prevent these problems by using care strategies believed to minimise or avoid trauma. Studies that have examined rates of perineal trauma demonstrate considerable variation in rates of laceration and the use of episiotomy. This variation has been recorded between hospital centres (North West Thames Region 1993; South East Thames Region 1995) and between individual midwives (Wilkerson 1984). Between-country variation is also observed in pooled population statistics; for example, in the USA, 50 per cent of women who have a vaginal birth also have an episiotomy (Albers *et al* 1996b), whereas in England, Wales and France around 30 per cent of women experience this intervention (Mascarenhas *et al* 1992). Factors likely to influence this variation include whether or not episiotomy is considered an appropriate routine intervention in normal labour, and the skill and experience of the practitioner involved with the delivery (Sleep *et al* 1989).

Interventions advocated to try to maintain the integrity of the perineal body include the direct application of oils, such as almond or olive, to massage or stretch the perineum. So far, published evidence from the small trials assessing perineal massage has failed to produce convincing evidence on which to base practice (Avery & Burket 1986; Avery & Van Arsdale 1987; Labrecque *et al* 1994). The application of hot and cold compresses is also promoted by some. An observational cohort study of over 3000 women carried out in the USA (Albers *et al* 1996b) analysed predetermined items of information selected from the routine records for every woman who gave birth in the three participating nurse-midwifery centres during a 12-month period. From these data, the researchers identified a statistically significant reduction in perineal trauma among women whose midwives reported using warm compresses during second stage. Women who had had oils or lubricants applied to the perineum were reported to have a statistically significant increase in perineal trauma. It is important to acknowledge that, because women were not randomly assigned to care in this study, there may be alternative explanations for the results. It is therefore not possible to be sure whether the outcomes observed are as a result of the interventions concerned or of some other factor. However, these findings are particularly useful in highlighting questions that need to be asked in prospective randomised controlled studies.

Several different approaches to perineal management involving varying levels of manual intervention have been described (Floud 1994a, 1994b). Supporting or 'guarding' the perineum is a widespread practice in which the midwife applies direct pressure to the woman's perineum throughout contractions during the second stage. The purpose is to maintain the integrity of the perineal tissues by avoiding abrupt rupture caused by the pressure of the baby's head. At the same time, the midwife may exert gentle pressure on the baby's head in an attempt to maintain flexion and to control it as it crowns. Lateral flexion is then used to facilitate delivery of the shoulders. These components comprise a 'hands-on' method of perineal management. Some midwives modify the 'hands-on' method and advocate digital control of the fetal head during crowning without guarding the perineum. In contrast, others may use a 'hands poised' method in which the midwife does not touch the perineum or baby's head. There are firm advocates for all of these approaches, but there is as yet no reliable general-isable evidence on which to base practice.

A large randomised controlled trial to compare the 'hands-on' with the 'hands poised' method is ongoing (HOOP Study Collaborative Group, 1994, unpublished protocol). The primary outcome to be assessed is perineal pain at 10 days after delivery, and women who take part are also being asked about other physical outcomes (for example, dyspareunia and incontinence) at 3 months after birth. The results of this study will be available in 1998 and will help midwives and childbearing women to make informed decisions about the effects of these techniques.

■ The use of episiotomy

An episiotomy is a surgical incision into the perineum designed to enlarge the vulval outlet and (apart from cutting the umbilical cord) is the most commonly performed operation in obstetrics (Cunningham *et al* 1989). Its purpose is either to facilitate birth as quickly as possible or to minimise or control perineal trauma. As with any surgical intervention, there should be clear indications that the procedure is necessary.

It has been suggested that specific maternal benefits of the routine use of episiotomy could include prevention of damage to the anal sphincter and pelvic floor muscles, and the principal fetal benefit would be to reduce trauma to the fetal head (Thacker & Banta 1983). The risks of such a procedure include excessive bleeding, an increased potential for infection and spontaneous extension to involve the anal sphincter and rectal mucosa (Thorp *et al* 1987).

Where fetal indications are clear, such as cases in which there is fetal distress and it is therefore essential to expedite delivery, there is little argument for withholding an episiotomy. However, there is controversy about the appropriate maternal indications for episiotomy.

A number of studies have compared liberal and restricted uses of episiotomy for normal vaginal birth in different practice settings (Harrison *et al* 1984; House *et al* 1986; Sleep *et al* 1984; Klein *et al* 1992; Argentine Episiotomy Trial Collaborative Group 1993). None has demonstrated that liberal, compared with restricted, use confers benefit on the mother in terms of the degree of perineal trauma sustained or subsequent outcomes such as maternally reported pain and discomfort at 10 days and 3 months after birth, or in the rates of dyspareunia.

The largest randomised controlled trial of alternative episiotomy policies (Argentine Episiotomy Trial Collaborative Group 1993) involved 2606 women (60 per cent of whom were nulliparous) in uncomplicated, term labour who were randomised to a policy of either selective or routine medio-lateral episiotomy. As with previous studies (Sleep *et al* 1984; Klein *et al* 1992), the selective or restricted policy required that the attending clinician should attempt to avoid using an episiotomy, and restrict its use to fetal indications only and the liberal policy involved attempting to prevent a tear. Anterior perineal trauma was more commonly noted in the selective episiotomy group (19 per cent compared with 8 per cent) and posterior trauma requiring repair was more common in the routine group (63 per cent compared with 88 per cent).

In a large trial evaluating the routine and liberal use of median episiotomy conducted in Canada (Klein *et al* 1992), severe perineal trauma, that is, trauma involving the anal sphincter and rectal mucosa, was found to be more commonly associated with the routine use of episiotomy.

Given that no significant difference between the liberal and routine use of episiotomy has been identified in neonatal outcome in terms of Apgar score or the number of babies requiring admission to a special care baby unit (Sleep *et al* 1984; Klein *et al* 1992), and that no maternal benefits have been found for liberal use, accumulating evidence provides convincing grounds for challenging the routine use of episiotomy for women in normal, term labour.

■ Midline versus medio-lateral episiotomy

Although medio-lateral episiotomy is widely used in many parts of the world and is the procedure evaluated in all but one of the trials described above (the exception being Klein *et al* 1992), midline or median episiotomy is the norm in some countries. A medio-lateral incision is the technique most commonly used in the UK and is designed to avoid damage to the Bartholin's gland and the anal sphincter. Median episiotomy, carried out along the natural line of insertion of the perineal muscles, is used extensively in North America, its proponents believing that it confers benefit in terms of a reduction in the risk of extension and of ease of repair (Sleep 1993) compared with medio-lateral episiotomy.

To date, only one small controlled study involving 356 women has directly compared the use of median with medio-lateral episiotomy (Coats *et al* 1980). Although the investigators sought randomly to assign women to one or other episiotomy technique, allocation was determined according to the last digit on a woman's case note number. It was therefore possible to predict which technique would be allocated, and this raises the possibility of selection bias. In fact, the results showed that more women who had forceps or breech deliveries were assigned to the medio-lateral group than would have been expected to be allocated to this group by chance. This may have been because practitioners taking part in the trial were more confident and competent in using medio-lateral episiotomy and thus did not wish to allocate the less familiar technique to women whom they considered at greater risk of perineal trauma and pain. In addition, a substantial number of women who were randomised in the trial were excluded from the final analysis because they did not receive the allocated episiotomy technique. This means that the results were not based on the policies as randomised and may therefore have been subject to further bias. Because of these flaws in the evaluation, it is not possible to make any recommendation for practice in the light of these results. The absence of good-quality research means that the choice of midline or medio-lateral episiotomy continues to be influenced by personal practitioner preferences and local policies rather than any robust evidence.

■ Recommendations for clinical practice in the light of currently available evidence

1. Arbitrarily limiting the length of the second stage of labour for all women is likely to subject some to inappropriate interventions and therefore cause more harm than good. If labour is progressing and there are no signs of maternal or fetal problems, the observation that the second stage is 'long' is not, of itself, an indication for active intervention.

2. The care of women who experience precipitate delivery has not been subject to evaluation and therefore remains an area in which pragmatic practice and custom prevail. The principles of management are to remain with the woman to comfort and support her, and to try to control the birth of the baby's head as much as possible to minimise sudden expulsion, with a concomitant risk of cerebral trauma for the newborn and perineal laceration for the mother. Further research is required to determine the most effective care.

3. There is good evidence that adopting a dorsal position induces maternal aortocaval compression and consequent hypotension, which in turn compromises fetal oxygen levels. These effects are likely to be potentiated by a prolonged adoption of this position and by conventional epidural anaesthetic. Further research is required to establish whether or not there are significant differences between different birth positions in terms of neonatal or maternal outcome.

4. There is no convincing evidence that the use of an upright position in itself increases the risk of a clinically important blood loss or any other serious maternal or neonatal morbidity. However, restricting the position a woman is able to adopt so that she is unable to change position when she wishes may be associated with such unwanted outcomes.

5. Organised pushing involves encouraging a woman to hold her breath for several seconds. This increases maternal intrathoracic pressure and initially raises and then lowers blood pressure, so that fetal oxygenation may be reduced. These changes seem not be important if the baby is healthy but may lead to morbidity if the fetus is already compromised or if maternal effort is prolonged. In the light of the available evidence, 'organised' pushing does not offer any benefit over

supporting and enabling spontaneous maternal effort for women who are not using an epidural anaesthetic.

6. Organised pushing may be appropriately used to assist women who have an effective epidural anaesthetic during the second stage of labour. There is no evidence to suggest that encouraging these women to bear down as soon as full dilatation is diagnosed is more effective than waiting until the vertex is visible at the introitus.

7. Perineal care, such as the direct application of oils to massage or stretch the perineum and the application of hot and cold compresses, remains inadequately evaluated. It is not possible to recommend the widespread use of such techniques until they have been more rigorously tested.

8. There are several different perineal management techniques involving varying levels of manual intervention. None has yet been adequately evaluated and there is thus no reliable information on which to base practice; one large randomised controlled trial is currently comparing two commonly used techniques.

9. Where fetal indications are clear, such as cases in which there is fetal distress and it is therefore essential to expedite delivery, it is appropriate to carry out an episiotomy.

10. Given that no significant difference between liberal and routine uses of episiotomy has been identified in terms of neonatal outcome and no maternal benefits have been found for liberal use, accumulating evidence provides convincing grounds for challenging the routine use of episiotomy for women in normal, term labour. The comparison of medio-lateral and median episiotomy is long overdue.

■ Practice check

- Does your practice area have guidelines stating an upper time limit for the duration of the second stage of labour? If so, are the guidelines based on recent evidence and are they appropriately referenced?

- What are the practice guidelines for women who have an epidural during the second stage? Can these women adopt a lateral or semi-recumbent position? When is a woman with an effective epidural directed to start pushing?

- What proportion of women (without an epidural anaesthetic) give birth in your practice area in a position other than semirecumbent? Are women encouraged to change position freely during labour? Is there a range of physical aids (such as beanbags and rocking chairs) to assist this?

- How often do you carry out an episiotomy? Are records kept about the reasons for episiotomy? If so, do you and your colleagues review these records regularly?

- Would you say that you usually direct or organise pushing for a woman? What do your colleagues do? During antenatal classes, are women told to expect that the midwife will take the lead and instruct them to push?

☐ Acknowledgements

I am grateful to my colleagues at the National Perinatal Epidemiology Unit in Oxford, most especially those working on the HOOP Study, for their help and support, and to Jennifer Sleep, Professor in Nursing and Midwifery Research at Thames Valley University, whose unparalleled contribution and commitment to research evidence about second-stage midwifery care provided the basis for this chapter.

■ References

Albers LL, Schiff M, Gorwoda JG 1996a The length of active labor in normal pregnancies. Obstetrics and Gynecology 87(3): 355–9

Albers LL, Anderson D, Cragin L *et al* 1996b Factors leading to perineal trauma in childbirth. Journal of Nurse-Midwifery 41(4): 269–76

Aldrich CJ, D'Antona D, Spencer JAD *et al* 1995a The effect of maternal posture on fetal cerebral oxygenation during labour. British Journal of Obstetrics and Gynaecology 102: 14–19

Aldrich CJ, D'Antona D, Spencer JAD 1995b The effect of maternal pushing on fetal oxygenation and blood volume during the second stage of labour. British Journal of Obstetrics and Gynaecology 102: 448–53

Argentine Episiotomy Trial Collaborative Group 1993 Routine vs selective episiotomy: a randomized controlled trial. Lancet 342: 1517–18

Avery MD, Burket BA 1986 Effect of perineal massage on the incidence of episiotomy and perineal laceration in a nurse-midwifery service. Journal of Nurse-Midwifery 31(3): 128–34

Avery MD, Van Arsdale L 1987 Perineal massage: effect on the incidence of episiotomy and laceration in a nulliparous population. Journal of Nurse-Midwifery 32(3): 181–4

Bassell GM, Humayan SG, Marx GF (1980) Maternal bearing down efforts – another fetal risk? Obstetrics and Gynecology 56: 39–41

Chan DPC 1963 Positions during labour. British Medical Journal 1: 100–2

Coats PM, Chan KK, Wikins M, Beard RJ 1980 A comparison between midline and mediolateral episiotomies. British Journal of Obstetrics and Gynaecology 87: 408–12

Crowley P, Elbourne D, Ashurst H, Garcia J, Murphey D, Duigan N 1991 Delivery in an obstetric birth chair: a randomized controlled trial. British Journal of Obstetrics and Gynaecology 98: 667–74

Cunningham FG, MacDonald PC, Gant NF 1989 Conduct of normal labor and delivery. In Williams Obstetrics, 18th edn. Prentice Hall, London, Ch 16, p323

Dunham C, Myers F, Barnden N, McDougall A, Kelly TL, Aria B 1991 Mamatoto: a celebration of birth. Virago, London, pp99–101

Floud E 1994a Protecting the perineum in childbirth, 1, A retrospective view. British Journal of Midwifery 2: 258–63

Floud E 1994b Protecting the perineum in childbirth, 3, Perineal care today. British Journal of Midwifery 2: 359–60

Freidman EA 1955 Primigravid labor: a graphicostatistical analysis. Obstetrics and Gynecology 6(6): 567–88

Freidman EA 1956 Labor in multiparas: a graphicostatistical analysis. Obstetrics and Gynecology 8(6): 691–703

Garcia J, Garforth S 1989 Labour and delivery routines in English consultant maternity units. Midwifery 5: 155–62

Garcia J, Garforth S, Ayers S 1986 Midwives confined? Labour ward policies and routines. Research and the Midwife Conference Proceedings, University of Manchester, pp74–80

Gardosi J, Hutson N, Lynch CB 1989 Randomised controlled trial of squatting in the second stage of labour. Lancet 2: 74–7

Gareberg B, Magnusson B, Sultan B, Wennerholm U-B, Wennergren M, Hagberg H (1994) Birth in standing position: a high frequency of third degree tears. Acta Obstetricia et Gynecologica Scandanavica 73: 630–3

Glazener CMA, Abdalla M, Stroud P, Naji S, Templeton A, Russell AT 1995 Postnatal morbidity: extent, causes, prevention and treatment. British Journal of Obstetrics and Gynaecology 102: 282–7

Halldorsdóttir S, Karlsdóttir SI 1996 Journeying through labour and delivery: perceptions of women who have given birth. Midwifery 12: 48–61

Harrison RF, Brennan M, North PM, Reed JV, Wickham EA 1984 Is routine episiotomy necessary? British Medical Journal 288: 1971–75

Hodnett ED 1995 Support from caregivers during childbirth. In Neilson JP, Crowther CA, Hodnett ED, Hofmyer GJ, Keirse MJNC, Renfrew MJ (eds) Pregnancy and childbirth module of the Cochrane Database of Systematic Reviews, issue 2. BMJ Publishing, London

HOOP Study Collaborative Group 1994 The randomized controlled trial of care of the perineum at delivery: hands on or poised? The HOOP Study. Unpublished protocol, National Perinatal Epidemiology Unit, Oxford

House MJ, Cario G, Jones MH 1986 Episiotomy and the perineum: a random controlled trial. Journal of Obstetrics and Gynaecology 7: 107–10

Humphrey M, Hounslow D, Morgan S, Wood C 1973 The influence of maternal posture at birth on the fetus. Journal of Obstetrics and Gynaecology of the British Commonwealth 80: 1075–80

Johnstone FD, Aboelmagd MS, Harouny AK 1987 Maternal posture in second stage and fetal acid base status. British Journal of Obstetrics and Gynaecology 94: 753–7

Kitzinger S 1991 Homebirth and other alternatives to hospital. Dorling Kindersley, London, pp153–4

Klein MC, Gauthier RJ, Jorgensen SH et al 1992 Does episiotomy prevent perineal trauma and pelvic floor relaxation? Online Journal of Clinical Trials 10

Knauth DG, Haloburdo EP 1986 Effect of pushing techniques in birthing chair on length of second stage of labour. Nursing Research 35(1): 49–51

Kurtz CS, Schneider H, Huch R, Huch A 1982 The influence of maternal position on the fetal transcutaneous oxygen pressure (tcpO2). Journal of Perinatal Medicine 10(supplement 2): 74–5

Labrecque M, Marcoux S, Pinault J-J, Laroche C, Martin S (1994) Prevention of perineal trauma by perineal massage during pregnancy: a pilot study. Birth 21: 20–5

McManus TJ, Calder AA 1978 Upright posture and the efficiency of labour. Lancet 1: 72–4

Mascarenhas L, Eliot BW, Mackenzie IZ 1992 A comparison of perineal outcome, antenatal and intrapartum care between England and Wales and France. British Journal of Obstetrics and Gynaecology 88: 955–8

Meticoglou SM, Manning F, Harman C, Morrison I 1995 Perinatal outcome in relation to second-stage duration. American Journal of Obstetrics and Gynecology 173(3): 906–12

Nikodem VC 1995a Upright versus recumbent position during second stage of labour. In Enkin MW, Keirse MJNC, Renfrew MJ, Neilson JP (eds) Pregnancy and childbirth module of the Cochrane Database of Systematic Reviews, issue 2. BMJ Publishing, London

Nikodem VC 1995b Early versus late pushing with epidural anaesthesia in 2nd stage of labour. In Enkin MW, Keirse MJNC, Renfrew MJ, Neilson JP (eds) Pregnancy and childbirth module of the Cochrane Database of Systematic Reviews, issue 2. BMJ Publishing, London

North West Thames Region 1993 North West Thames Region annual maternity figures 1992. St Mary's Maternity Information System, London, pp57–9

Parnell C, Roos-Langhoff J, Iversen R, Damgaard P 1993 Pushing method in the expulsive phase of labor. Acta Obstetricia et Gynecologica Scandinavica 72:31–5

Roberts JE, Goldstein SA, Gruener SJ, Maggio M, Mendez-Bauer C 1987 A descriptive analysis of involuntary bearing down efforts during the expulsive phase of labor. Journal of Obstetric, Gynaecological and Neonatal Nursing 16: 48–55

Saunders NSG, Paterson CM, Wadsworth J 1992 Neonatal and maternal morbidity in relation to the length of the second stage of labour. British Journal of Obstetrics and Gynaecology 96(5): 381–5

Sleep JM 1993 Physiology and management of the second stage of labour. In Bennett RV, Brown LK (eds) Myles' Textbook for midwives, 12th edn. Churchill Livingstone, London, Ch 14, pp210–12

Sleep JM, Grant A 1987 West Berkshire perineal management trial: three year follow-up. British Medical Journal 295: 749–51

Sleep JM, Grant A, Garcia J, Elbourne D, Spencer J, Chalmers I 1984 West Berkshire perineal management trial. British Medical Journal 289: 587–90

Sleep JM, Roberts J, Chalmers I 1989 Care during the second stage of labour. In Chalmers I, Enkin M, Kierse MJNC (eds) Effective care in pregnancy and childbirth. Oxford University Press, Oxford, Ch 66, pp1131, 1136

South East Thames Region 1995 Perinatal profile: a review of South East Thames perinatal statistics from 1988–89. STRHA, Bexhill-on-Sea, pp31–2

Stewart P 1991 Influence of posture in labour. Contemporary Reviews in Obstetrics and Gynaecology 3(3): 152–7

Stewart P, Spiby H 1989 A randomized study of sitting position for delivery using a newly designed obstetric chair. British Journal of Obstetrics and Gynaecology 96(3): 327–33

Stewart P, Hillan E, Calder AA 1983 A randomised trial to evaluate the use of a birth chair for delivery. Lancet 1: 1296–8

Sweet B 1992 Baillière's midwives dictionary, 8th edn. Baillière Tindall, London, p279

Thacker SE, Banta HD 1983 Benefits and risks of episiotomy; an interpretative review of the English language literature, 1860–1980. Obstetrical and Gynaecological Survey 38: 322–38

Thomson AM 1993 Pushing techniques in the second stage of labour. Journal of Advanced Nursing 18: 171–7

Thomson AM 1995 Maternal behaviour during spontaneous and directed pushing in second stage of labour. Journal of Advanced Nursing 22: 1027–34

Thorp JM, Bowes WA, Brame RG, Cefal R 1987 Selected use of midline episiotomy: effect on perineal trauma. Obstetrics and Gynaecology 70: 260–2
Turner MJ, Romney ML, Webb JB, Gordon H 1986 The birthing chair: an obstetric hazard? Journal of Obstetrics and Gynaecology 6: 232–5
United Kingdom Central Council for Nursing, Midwifery and Health Visiting 1993 Midwives rules. UKCC, London, p20
Waldenstrom U, Gottvall K 1991 A randomized trial of birthing stool or conventional semirecumbent position for second-stage labor. Birth 18: 5–10
Wilkerson VA 1984 The use of episiotomy in normal delivery. Midwives Chronicle and Nursing Notes 97: 106–10
Williams J 1993 Prolonged pregnancy and disorders of uterine action. In Bennet RV, Brown LK (eds) Myles' Textbook for midwives, 12th edn. Churchill Livingstone, London, Ch 25, pp389–99

■ Suggested further reading

Cochrane Library, The Cochrane Collaboration. Oxford Update Software/BMJ Publishing Group, London
MIDIRS/NHS Centre for Reviews and Dissemination 1996 Positions in labour and delivery: informed choice for professionals. MIDIRS, Bristol
Sleep J, Roberts J, Chalmers I 1989 Care during the second stage of labour. In Chalmers I, Enkin M, Kierse M (eds) Effective care in pregnancy and childbirth. Oxford University Press, Oxford, pp1129–44

Chapter 8

The third stage of labour

Juliet Wood and Jane Rogers

The third stage of labour begins with the birth of the baby and ends with the delivery of the placenta and membranes, a process which, for most women, is rapidly accomplished without complication. However, history testifies to the drama which can arise where problems, notably postpartum haemorrhage (PPH) occur, and contemporary midwifery textbooks still carry warnings similar to that published in 1718 by the apothecary, Nicholas Culpeper:

> A Woman cannot be said to be safely delivered, tho' the Child be born, till the After-burden be also taken from her... Women have an After-labour which sometimes proves more difficult than the first.

■ It is assumed that you are already aware of the following:

- The physiology of the third stage;
- The action and side-effects of ergometrine, Syntocinon and Syntometrine;
- Factors that increase the risk of primary PPH;
- The policy or guidelines in your place of work for third-stage management and the reasons given for them.

■ Complications of the third stage of labour

A recent report from UNICEF (1996) estimates that 585 000 women die from complications in childbirth every year, the majority being in the poorer parts of the world. In addition to this appalling figure, UNICEF suggests that, for every death, 30 more mothers are left with permanent disability or injury. Haemorrhage is known to be among the leading causes of maternal death (WHO 1996), and it is therefore not surprising that debate continues to rage over the best way to deal with the third stage of labour, given its attendant risks. There is a growing body of research evidence to inform the debate, and this chapter analyses the current state of the art, with a particular emphasis on the following questions:

- When is it appropriate to use drugs in the third stage?

- Which drugs are the most suitable for particular circumstances?

- What is the contribution of other elements, such as maternal effort, controlled cord traction (CCT) and maternal position?

■ Physiological management

Physiological management is the delivery of the placenta and membranes by maternal effort without the use of drugs. An overview undertaken by Prendiville *et al* (1988a) examines data from nine controlled trials from 1951 onwards in which an oxytocic drug was compared with either a placebo or no routine prophylactic in the management of the third stage of labour. The conclusion of the overview was that the routine use of oxytocic drugs increases the risk of provoking hypertension, but reduces the risk of PPH by about 40 per cent. The practical implication of this is that, for every 22 women given an oxytocic, one PPH is prevented. The advantages of giving an oxytocic must also be considered, together with the risk of rare but serious maternal morbidity (cardiac arrest, pulmonary oedema or intracerebral haemorrhage), which has been linked with oxytocic administration. Prendiville *et al* (1988a) conclude that the known benefits of routine oxytocic administration outweigh the likely risks in women who are not at increased cardiovascular risk.

The trials reviewed by Prendiville *et al* (1988a) spanned a period of 34 years, and the sample sizes ranged from 26 to 1459 women. A wide variety of oxytocic drugs was used, and there was a considerable range in the timing of their administration. Criteria for trial entry were not consistent, and a number of women entered were at high risk of PPH. Details were rarely documented of how the third stage was managed, including those aspects of management that may become necessary as the third stage proceeds, such as early cord clamping, giving of a therapeutic oxytocic drug, CCT and altering the woman's position. These 'piecemeal' elements might have their own significance within both the physiological and active management 'packages'. Gyte (1994) suggests that a more balanced review of the evidence could have been presented had the clinical impressions of the various researchers also been reported.

A recent meta-analysis undertaken by Prendiville and Elbourne (1995) includes three trials that involved women deemed to be at low risk of haemorrhage (Prendiville *et al* 1988b; Begley 1990; Thiliganathan 1992). This analysis shows that active management of the third stage of labour reduces maternal postpartum blood loss but increases nausea, vomiting, headache and hypertension. The trial undertaken by Thiliganathan (1992) was very small, but the remaining two trials are discussed in more detail below.

The Bristol Third Stage Trial, conducted by Prendiville *et al* (1988b), was a randomised controlled trial comparing active with physiological management. The policy of active management practised in this trial made a statistically significant difference to the following: it reduced the incidence of PPH (defined as a blood loss equal to or greater than 500 ml) from 17.9 per cent to 5.9 per cent; it shortened the third stage from 15 to 5 minutes; and it resulted in a reduced neonatal packed cell volume. There was also a greater need for therapeutic oxytocics in the physiological group (29.7 per cent versus 6.4 per cent). There were no significant differences in the incidence of neonatal jaundice or respiratory problems. Many women allocated to the physiological group had piecemeal management; in fact, less than half of this group actually achieved 'pure' physiological management. It is difficult to interpret the results of a trial in which there is a large deviation from the set protocol. However, a secondary analysis, looking only at the women who had actually received the management to which they had been allocated, showed that active management was still beneficial. A further drawback of the trial was that it allowed for the inclusion of women deemed to be at high risk of PPH. Acknowledging this, the authors made a further secondary analysis using data from only those women thought to be 'low risk', and there were still more adverse outcomes occurring in the physiological than the active group. A third problem in this trial was that few of the midwives involved in the study were experienced in carrying out physiological management, and the women in the physiological group may therefore have been at a disadvantage (Harding *et al* 1989). The authors recommended testing the same hypothesis in a setting where physiological management of the third stage was commonly practised by all midwives.

A further randomised controlled trial comparing active with physiological management, known as the Dublin Trial, was carried out by Begley (1990) and involved women thought to be at low risk of PPH. This is the only trial in which information on long-term sequelae (up to 6 weeks postpartum) has been collected. Statistically significant results were found for several outcomes; the incidence of PPH was higher in the physiological group, but there was a higher incidence of manual removal of placenta, secondary PPH and side-effects of ergometrine (nausea, headache and severe afterpains) in the actively managed group. The principal problem with this study is that the oxytocic (used either prophylactically or therapeutically) was ergometrine, administered intravenously. Although this management was in common use in this particular hospital at the time, this was not the case in most hospitals in England (Garcia *et al* 1987), so the results have limited generalisability. Piecemeal management occurred to a considerable degree in the group allocated to physiological management. The trial demonstrated that a PPH of 500–750 ml does not appear to cause problems for normal healthy women, and this raises the question of the clinical signif-

icance of an estimated blood loss under 750 ml and, in particular, the usefulness of the definition of PPH as used in the UK. Begley (1990) acknowledges
the problem that many of the midwives in the study were inexperienced in
physiological management. There is also a need to investigate whether it is
preferable to resort to the full range of components of active management
(rather than a piecemeal approach) when there is a need to interrupt the
physiological process, such as when the cord is round the neck and needs to
be clamped and cut early.

A trial set up at Hinchingbrooke Hospital in Huntingdon by the authors
aims to answer three main questions. First, it addresses the problem
previously mentioned of midwives being inexperienced in conducting a
physiological third stage. The midwives at Hinchingbrooke are experienced
in physiological management, so it is possible that differences in outcome
between the two groups will not be as great as in previous studies. Second,
recent studies suggest that adopting an upright posture for delivery may
predispose women to greater blood loss (Spiby 1991). In the two trials
already described, the women in the physiological group have been encouraged to deliver the placenta in a position aiding gravity; it is therefore
possible that the differences in blood loss between physiological and active
managements are a result of posture rather than other elements of expectant
management. This problem is being addressed in the Hinchingbrooke study
by randomising women to one of four groups in which both position and
third-stage management are prescribed. Third, the question of the clinical
relevance of blood loss will be addressed.

Gyte (1992) argues that a PPH is not necessarily dangerous for healthy
women delivered in a hospital setting; it is possible that physiological
management, although more hazardous in the short term, may be advanta-
geous in the longer term. The Hinchingbrooke trial takes into account
outcomes relating to maternal morbidity, such as fatigue and depression, and
problems associated with bleeding or uterine infection in the puerperium. The
hypothesis being tested is that active management of the third stage of labour
reduces the incidence of PPH even in a setting where both managements are
routinely practised for women thought to be at low risk of haemorrhage. A
total of 1512 took part in this randomised controlled trial in a district general
hospital between June 1993 and December 1995. Besides the primary
hypothesis, 16 other outcomes are being measured. Criteria for entry into the
trial excluded those at high risk of PPH, and mothers were excluded from the
study for the following reasons:

- Placenta praevia;

- A previous PPH;

- An antepartum haemorrhage after 20 weeks;

- Less than 32 completed weeks of pregnancy;

- Parity >4;

- Uterine fibroids;

- Anticoagulation therapy in pregnancy;

- Anaemia (haemoglobin level <10 g/dl);

- A non-cephalic presentation;

- Multiple pregnancy;

- Intrauterine death;

- Epidural anaesthesia;

- A Syntocinon drip for induction or augmentation;

- Intended instrumental or operative delivery;

- Any other circumstances in which the clinician feels that there were overwhelming contraindications to any of the managements.

A more detailed description of the method used can be found in the Midwifery Research Database (MIRIAD) (McCormick & Renfrew 1996).

☐ Issues raised by the Hinchingbrooke Third Stage Trial

The results of the Hinchingbrooke trial will be available in the second half of 1997. A number of interesting issues that are worthy of comment have evolved from this study. The first is that a significant number of eligible women chose not to take part in the study because they already had a preference for one or other management. Approximately one quarter of the total number of women delivering took part in the trial. Of those who did not take part, just over half were excluded for obstetric reasons, and a further quarter declined to take part because they wanted to exercise personal choice (as they would have done prior to commencement of the study). Their choices were made on the basis of little substantive evidence but, we suspect, of considerably more information than they would have received before the profile of third-stage management was so markedly raised by the trial. Approximately two-thirds of this group chose physiological management and one third active management. It is clear that there is a sizeable number of women who progress without intervention up to the birth of their babies and who wish to continue with a natural labour if this is an ' option presented to them. It is possible that this also demonstrates the extent to which many women wish to be partners in their care and to share in the responsibility of decision making. This consideration needs to be taken seriously by policy makers in the light of the underlying philosophy of the *Changing childbirth* report (DoH 1993) and its emphasis on client involvement in care.

Having focused on the group that chose not to be involved, it would be fair to say that we were constantly encouraged by the enthusiasm of the mothers who did take part. The rate of return for all the questionnaires was extremely high, 95 per cent of participants returning the questionnaire 6 weeks after delivery, and the comments elicited from the women regarding their experience of participating in the trial were, on the whole, very positive.

There was good adherence to the protocol on the part of the midwives, two-thirds of the group assigned to physiological management actually receiving it. This is a much higher proportion than in the recent studies (Begley 1990; Prendiville *et al* 1988b) and presumably reflects the confidence and experience of the midwives in physiological management of the third stage of labour. Enthusiasm on the part of the staff was extremely encouraging and was essential to the smooth running of the project. At the beginning and end of the trial, the midwives filled in questionnaires considering their views of research and third stage management. This information will be interesting to explore with regard to the individual midwife's experience in a physiological third stage, a subject raised for further research by the authors of the Bristol trial (Prendiville *et al* 1988b).

☐ The Lente trial

A similar trial to that taking place in Hinchingbrooke is the Lente trial (Buitendijk *et al* 1995), which also compares active with physiological management. This has been instigated and carried out by midwives in Holland, and the results are eagerly awaited. The setting of the study is different from that of the Hinchingbrooke trial because all the mothers in the trial give birth at home. In addition, the oxytocic being investigated is Syntocinon 5 IU given intramuscularly. Like the Hinchingbrooke study, the sample is made up of women at low risk of PPH and there is postpartum follow-up, in this case at 3 months after the birth. Obviously, when reported, these results will have to be interpreted in the light of the differences in the population studied, compared with those in the other trials, and the unique organisation of care in the Netherlands.

■ Active management of the third stage

In their survey of policies and practice in maternity units in England and Wales, Garcia *et al* (1987) found that the vast majority of maternity units had, at that time, a policy of using active management of the third stage for all women. This is generally defined as being composed of three elements, namely the giving of a drug (either an oxytocin or an ergot derivative), the clamping and cutting of the umbilical cord and the use of traction on the cord to hasten delivery of the placenta and membranes. Of these three elements, cutting and clamping of the cord has, in the main, gone unchallenged in the literature since it is widely accepted that the artificial contraction induced by the drug could otherwise lead to a sudden overtransfusion of blood to the baby (Inch 1989; Sleep 1993). However, the results of one trial (Oxford Midwives Research Group 1991) counter this argument, demonstrating no clear evidence for the benefit of early cord clamping.

☐ Drugs

There is no doubt that the use of drugs in the third stage of labour has been instrumental in reducing the rate of deaths from PPH over the past 50 years in Britain (DoH 1996), although it is impossible to separate out the relative contribution afforded in this context by other developments such as blood transfusion and antibiotics.

In active management of the third stage, the clinician must decide which drug to give, in what dose, by which route and when. The first drug to be used was ergot of rye, whose pharmacological properties were suspected from observations of the high rate of miscarriage among women who worked in the rye fields in the early 19th century. It was originally used to stem PPH and to augment prolonged labour (with sometimes drastic consequences for both mother and baby). Ergometrine was isolated in 1935 by Dudley and Moir and was available in intramuscular and intravenous forms by the late 1940s. Until then, its use (in the form of powders, tinctures, infusions and so on) in relation to the third stage had been restricted to being given only after the placenta was delivered, for fear of its being trapped. However, texts since 1948 generally advocate its administration between the birth of the baby and the delivery of the placenta. (For a succinct summary of the history of the use of ergot, see Kerr *et al* 1954; also Tew 1993.) The oxytocic properties of posterior pituitary extract (pitocin or its modern equivalent oxytocin) had been realised in 1909 by Blair-Bell, but the two drugs were not combined until 1963 when the drug Syntometrine was successfully marketed on the grounds of uniting the advantages of both. According to the manufacturer's information leaflet, when the drug is used intramuscularly, tocograph recordings demonstrate the onset of uterine contractions within 2.5 minutes owing to the Syntocinon component, followed by a sustained tonic contraction at about 7 minutes as a result of the action of ergometrine. Although both its components are individually available for intravenous use, Syntometrine itself is not recommended by the manufacturers for intravenous use. The reason for this is not clear in the current information leaflet.

In 1988 the same team that undertook the overview of trials comparing active with physiological management, described earlier, published an overview of controlled trials comparing the effects of ergot alkaloids, prostaglandins, oxytocin and Syntometrine (Elbourne *et al* 1988). While acknowledging the limitations of the evidence available to them, the authors concluded that ergometrine alone did not have any advantage over Syntometrine in terms of reducing the risk of PPH and that it did, indeed, increase the risk of hypertension, especially when compared with oxytocin alone. They therefore advised that ergometrine should not be used routinely in management of the third stage. According to the same overview, the use of prostaglandins is still in its infancy, and the evidence relating to it is not, as yet, clinically applicable. The studies available in the late 1980s that compared oxytocin and Syntometrine were subject to considerable bias, and Elbourne *et al* (1988) were therefore cautious in their conclusions for clinical practice. They summarised the evidence by suggesting that Syntometrine is likely to reduce the risk of PPH but with possible adverse effects in terms of hypertension.

In line with their recommendation for more reliable evidence, there have subsequently been two large double-blind randomised controlled trials comparing Syntometrine (ergometrine 0.5 mg with Syntocinon 5 IU) with Syntocinon (10 IU), both being given by the intramuscular route. The first was an Australian trial involving 3497 women (McDonald *et al* 1993), and the second involving 992 women (Yuen *et al* 1995) was carried out in Hong Kong. In both studies, the estimated blood loss was lower in the group receiving Syntometrine, although this did not make a significant difference to the postnatal haemoglobin estimation at 24 hours (Yuen *et al* 1995) or 2 days (McDonald *et al* 1993), or to the need for blood transfusion. In the Australian study, it was noted that Syntometrine provided a small but clear protection against blood loss estimated at 1 litre or more. In clinical practice, it was suggested that this benefit would be relevant for between eight and 11 women per 1000. Since severe PPH is a rare phenomenon, the authors point out that this advantage needs to be balanced against the common short-term side-effects of nausea, vomiting and hypertension, which were much more marked in the Syntometrine group. Women in this group were seven times more likely to vomit and five times more likely to have a diastolic blood pressure greater than 100 mmHg than were those receiving oxytocin alone.

In contrast to these findings, and perhaps surprisingly given the well-documented hypertensive effects of ergometrine, the Hong Kong study did not find a significant difference in these side-effects. Despite the lack of evidence to demonstrate any detrimental effect from the higher estimated blood loss in the oxytocin group, Yuen *et al* (1995) recommended that Syntometrine should be the drug of choice, principally because they recorded a 40 per cent decrease in the need for a repeat oxytocic in the Syntometrine group. This difference was also noted to reach statistical significance in the Australian study, but, when analysed on the basis of the drug actually received (as opposed to on an intention-to-treat basis), the effect disappeared; similar analysis is not available in the Hong Kong study. The data relating to manual removal of the placenta are difficult to interpret since no definitions are given regarding the time elapsing before the placenta was deemed to be retained.

In summary, the evidence suggests that Syntometrine gives better protection for women at risk of severe PPH (blood loss >1000 ml) but may increase the risk of vomiting and hypertension in the whole population of newly delivered women. The decision about which oxytocic to use needs to take into account the relative consequences of these effects for the individual mother, which will depend, in part, on her general health and her obstetric history. Useful information could come from studying the relative effects of different doses of oxytocin (for example, 10 IU versus 20 IU) when used alone, as suggested by McDonald *et al* (1993), although oxytocin is at present not licensed for intramuscular use in the UK. In terms of route and timing for giving an oxytocic, there is as yet no evidence for guiding practice, and it is likely that the great majority of practitioners will continue to give the drugs intramuscularly with the delivery of the anterior shoulder or immediately following the birth of the baby.

☐ Clamping and cutting the umbilical cord

When an oxytocic drug has been administered, the birth attendant usually cuts and clamps the cord before the contraction induced by the oxytocic occurs. This theoretically protects the baby from a sudden transfusion of blood caused by an artificially strong contraction but also denies it the physiological transfer that would occur if the uterus were left to its own devices (Montgomery 1960; Yao & Lind 1974; Inch 1989; Oxford Midwives Research Group, 1991). There is a school of thought that advocates releasing the clamp from the maternal end in order to encourage the blood to drain away, thus reducing the bulkiness of the placenta, promoting the contraction and retraction of the uterine muscles and facilitating delivery (Botha 1968; Inch 1985). This requires care on the part of the midwife in order to avoid blood splashing, but, in the absence of contradictory research evidence, the theoretical basis suggests that it is a logical way to proceed. If, as has been suggested by Lapido (1972), early cord clamping increases the risk of isoimmunisation in Rhesus-negative women, this technique would also militate against this unwanted effect.

☐ Cord traction

The concept of pulling on the umbilical cord developed as a technique for avoiding the entrapment of the placenta by contraction of the uterus and closing of the cervix. It was used long before oxytocic drugs were employed and has persisted to this day; research by Spencer (1962) on CCT led to the method becoming widely used in this country. Various modifications to the technique have been advocated by different practitioners, and these relate to the position of the free hand (usually used to 'guard' the uterus) and the timing of the traction. There is a debate within the literature regarding the need to await signs of placental separation (the trickle of blood, the rising of the uterus and the lengthening of the cord) before applying traction. The proponents of waiting for these signs argue that this reduces the risk of uterine inversion and PPH (Bell 1946; Kerr *et al* 1954; Levy & Moore

1985). Levy and Moore (1985) studied the management of the third stage of 489 women who delivered normally. They found that waiting for placental separation increased the length of the third stage by approximately 1 minute. The PPH rate was significantly higher, at 15 per cent, when the midwife unsuccessfully attempted immediate CCT (without waiting for signs of separation and descent apart from contraction of the uterus) and then waited for a few minutes before reapplying traction. PPH rates were similar (about 5 per cent) in the group in which signs were awaited and in that in which immediate CCT was successful on the first attempt. On the strength of these findings, Levy and Moore (1985) advocate waiting for signs of separation and descent prior to CCT. However, as Levy (1990) acknowledges, this study was small and was open to selection bias; further research is recommended on the subject.

It is also possible to encourage the mother to push the placenta out herself once separation has occurred instead of using cord traction; indeed, this method may be necessary if the cord has started to tear and the remaining portion of cord is inaccessibly high in the vagina or uterus. She may be helped by having firm pressure applied over the lower part of her abdomen by the attendant's hand. This method requires cooperation and energy from the woman but avoids the risk of snapping the cord.

■ Postpartum haemorrhage

The difficulty of estimating the amount of blood shed at delivery is well recognised among researchers and clinicians alike (Brant 1967). While it is possible to set up artificial scenarios in which measured amounts of blood are distributed over drapes in order for midwives to practise estimation, it is more important for clinicians to recognise when blood loss is having an adverse effect on a woman since, for many different reasons, women seem to vary in their ability to tolerate a given blood loss. This fact has led to some authors (Levy 1990; Gyte 1994) questioning the usefulness of the 500 ml definition of PPH since, in countries where general health is good, few women are adversely affected by this volume of recorded blood loss. In Holland, it is generally accepted that blood loss of over 1 litre is a more useful working definition (Buitendijk *et al* 1995). Midwives should bear in mind that large blood losses are most commonly underestimated (Newton *et al* 1961; Levy 1990). In the Department of Health Report on Confidential Enquiries into Maternal Deaths in the United Kingdom 1988–1990 (DoH 1994), of 11 deaths attributed to PPH, only one followed a normal delivery (and this was a far from straightforward labour). In the latest report (DoH 1996), there were eight deaths in 3 years attributed to primary PPH, of which three followed normal uncomplicated deliveries. Two of these women declined blood transfusion, but in the other case it is not clear how the situation might have been avoided. It is absolutely essential that midwives are aware of the clear guidelines for the management of massive obstetric haemorrhage published in the 1994 report (DoH 1994) and the guidelines for the treatment of women who decline blood transfusion, discussed in the 1996 report (DoH 1996).

■ Recommendations for clinical practice in the light of currently available evidence

1. Unbiased information regarding the benefits and hazards of physiological and active management should be available for all pregnant women. Midwives should be fully conversant with the reasons for some women being more at risk of PPH than others and give information to mothers accordingly.

2. Opportunity for discussion about the third stage should be given to the mother before labour begins. If there are reasons during pregnancy or labour why her original plan for third-stage management should be changed, these should be discussed with her.

3. Conditional on the above points being achieved, the choice of third-stage management for women at low risk of PPH should be made by the mother and midwife together.

4. If there have been problems with the third stage in previous births, it is essential that as much information as possible is available and made clear in the mother's notes, particularly those carried by her. Other relevant information, such as the latest haemoglobin level result and blood pressure recordings in pregnancy, should also be conspicuously documented.

5. If physiological management is attempted but intervention in the form of an oxytocic drug is needed, for example in the event of a heavier than normal blood loss, management must proceed actively.

6. Active management of the third stage of labour is recommended for women at high risk of PPH.

7. If an oxytocic drug is to be given, the midwife should, where possible, take into account the relative risks of substantial PPH or increased blood pressure for that individual mother and choose the drug accordingly.

8. The mother's consent to the administration of an oxytocic should be obtained.

9. The midwife should be familiar with, and competent in, the initial action taken to control a PPH and in how to recognise the need to involve a medical practitioner. She should be conversant with the procedures undertaken in the medical management of a large PPH and be proficient in the special skills required. For example, it is wise for a

midwife attending home births (where medical aid may not be close at hand) to be proficient at siting an intravenous cannula.

10. Midwives considering the conduct of physiological third stage must do so in the light of Rule 40 of the *Midwives Rules* (UKCC 1993). This states in paragraph 2 that a practising midwife must not, except in an emergency, undertake any treatment that she has not been trained to give, either before or after registration as a midwife.

■ Practice check

- Are options for third stage management discussed with women in the antenatal period in your area? Do you think they should be?

- Having assessed their suitability, would you be competent to offer women physiological management of the third stage of labour and, if not, how do you intend to develop the necessary skills?

- Are you sufficiently familiar with the evidence on the different oxytocics to advise individual women on the best choice of oxytocic for them?

- What is the PPH rate in your place of work?

- Think through how you would prioritise your actions in the event of a large PPH if you were the only midwife in attendance.

☐ Acknowledgements

We would like to thank the staff of the National Perinatal Epidemiology Unit in Oxford, in particular Diana Elbourne, Rona McCandlish, Ann Truesdale and Sarah Ayers, for their unstinting support in the conduct of the Hinchingbrooke Third Stage Trial. Great credit is also due to the staff of the Hinchingbrooke Maternity Unit for their encouragement and hard work, and to the women who were so willing to help and participate.

■ References

Begley C 1990 A comparison of 'active' and 'physiological' management of the third stage of labour. Midwifery   6: 3–17
Bell A 1946 A pocket obstetrics. Churchill, London, pp88–9
Botha M 1968 The management of the umbilical cord in labour. South African Journal of Obstetrics and Gynaecology   6(2): 30–3
Brant H 1967 Precise estimation of postpartum haemorrhage: difficulties and importance. British Medical Journal   1: 398–400
Buitendijk S, Aitink M, vanDiem M, Herschderfer K 1995 The Lente trial – study into the routine administration of oxytocin in the third stage of labour in midwifery practice. Personal communication

Culpeper N 1718 Culpeper's Compleat and experienc'd midwife: in two parts, 3rd edn. London

Department of Health 1993 Changing childbirth. Report of the Expert Maternity Group. HMSO, London

Department of Health 1994 Report on confidential enquiries into maternal deaths in the United Kingdom 1988–1990. HMSO, London

Department of Health 1996 Report on confidential enquiries into maternal deaths in the United Kingdom 1991–1993. HMSO, London

Elbourne D, Prendiville W, Chalmers I 1988 Choice of oxytocic preparation for routine use in the management of the third stage of labour: an overview of the evidence from controlled trials. British Journal of Obstetrics and Gynaecology 95: 17–30

Garcia J, Garforth S, Ayers S 1987 The policy and practice of midwifery study: introduction and methods. Midwifery 3(1): 2–9

Gyte G 1992 The significance of blood loss at delivery. MIDIRS Midwifery Digest 2(1): 88–92

Gyte G 1994 Evaluation of the meta-analysis on the effects, on both mother and baby, of the various components of 'active' management of the third stage of labour. Midwifery 10: 183–99

Harding J, Elbourne D, Prendiville W 1989 Views of mothers and midwives participating in the Bristol randomized controlled trial of the management of the third stage of labour. Birth 16: 1–6

Inch S 1985 Management of the third stage of labour – another cascade of intervention? Midwifery 1: 114–22

Inch S 1989 Birthrights – a parents' guide to modern childbirth, 2nd edn. Green Print, London, Ch 7, pp145–91

Kerr J, Johnstone R, Phillips M 1954 Historical review of British obstetrics and gynaecology 1800–1950. Livingstone, London

Lapido O 1972 Management of the third stage of labour, with particular reference to reduction of feto–maternal transfusion. British Medical Journal 1: 721–3

Levy V 1990 The midwife's management of the third stage of labour. In Alexander J, Levy V, Roch S (eds) Intrapartum care: a research-based approach. Macmillan, London, p144

Levy V, Moore J 1985 The midwife's management of the third stage of labour. Nursing Times 81(39):47–50

McCormick F, Renfrew MJ (eds) 1996 The Midwifery Research Database (MIRIAD). Books for Midwives Press, Hale

McDonald S, Prendiville W, Blair E 1993 Randomized controlled trial of oxytocin alone versus oxytocin and ergometrine in active management of the third stage of labour. British Medical Journal 307: 1167–71

Montgomery T 1960 The umbilical cord. Clinical Obstetrics and Gynaecology 3: 900–10

Newton M, Mosey L, Egli G, Gifford W, Hull C 1961 Blood loss during and immediately after delivery. Obstetrics and Gynaecology 17(1): 9–18

Oxford Midwives Research Group 1991 A study of the relationship between the delivery to cord clamping interval and the time of cord separation. Midwifery 7: 167–76

Prendiville W, Elbourne D 1995 Active versus conservative third stage management – low risk women. In Keirse MJNC, Renfrew M, Neilson J, Crowther C (eds) Pregnancy and childbirth module of the Cochrane Pregnancy and Childbirth Database, issue 2. Available from BMJ Publishing Group, London

Prendiville W, Elbourne D, Chalmers I 1988a The effects of routine oxytocic administration in the management of the third stage of labour: an overview of the evidence from controlled trials. British Journal of Obstetrics and Gynaecology 95: 3–16

Prendiville W, Harding J, Elbourne D, Stirrat G 1988b The Bristol Third Stage Trial: active versus physiological management of the third stage of labour. British Medical Journal 297: 1295–300

Sleep J 1993 Physiology and management of the third stage of labour. In Bennett V, Brown L (eds) Myles' Textbook for midwives, 12th edn. Churchill Livingstone, Edinburgh, Ch 15

Spencer P 1962 Controlled cord traction in the management of the third stage of labour. British Medical Journal 1: 1728–32

Spiby H 1991 Upright v. recumbent position during second stage of labour. In Chalmers I (ed.) Oxford Database of Perinatal Trials, version 1.2, disk issue 6, Autumn, record 3335

Tew M 1993 Safer childbirth? A critical review of the history of maternity care, 3rd edn. Chapman & Hall, London

Thiliganathan B 1992 Management of the third stage of labour in women at low risk of postpartum haemorrhage. In Chalmers I (ed.) Oxford Database of Perinatal Trials, version 1.2, disk issue 7, Spring, record 6040

UNICEF 1996 The progress of nations. New evidence collated, 11 June, New York

United Kingdom Central Council for Nursing, Midwifery and Health Visiting 1993 Midwives Rules. Rule 40. UKCC, London, p20

World Health Organization 1996 The mother–baby package: an overview. WHO, Geneva

Yao A, Lind J 1974 Placental transfusion. American Diseases of Childhood 127: 128–41

Yuen P, Chan N, Yim S, Chang A 1995 A randomized double blind comparison of Syntometrine and Syntocinon in the management of the third stage of labour. British Journal of Obstetrics and Gynaecology 102: 377–80

■ Suggested further reading

Still D 1994 Postpartum haemorrhage and other problems of the third stage. In James D, Steer P, Weiner C, Gonik B (eds) High risk pregnancy: management options. WB Saunders, London

Chapter 9

Care in normal labour: a feminist perspective

Carol Bates

Childbirth is, in the Western world, no longer perceived as a normal, physiological process, even in women who are fit and healthy and have had an uncomplicated pregnancy. This is because, since the 1960s, childbirth has been 'managed' by obstetricians who consider that childbirth, in all women, can be considered normal only in retrospect (Savage 1986; Wertz & Wertz 1989). This has resulted in a steady rise in the use of fetal monitoring, induction, Syntocinon, epidural analgesia, episiotomy, forceps and caesarean section: childbirth is now 'medicalised'.

Oakley argues that the way in which childbirth is 'managed' affects the position of women in society (Oakley 1993: 127). Rich considers that the 'passive' suffering of childbirth is universally seen as a 'natural' female destiny, and unfortunately women do not realise that this passivity is then carried on into every sphere of the female life experience. Rich is of the view that childbirth controlled by men does not allow a woman to bring to it her own character, intelligence and instinctive and physical equipment (Rich 1977: 129).

The purpose of this chapter is to show how the involvement of men in childbirth, and the medicalisation of childbirth that has ensued, is not in the best interests of women or midwives. A feminist perspective will be used to discuss the concept of patriarchy and how it works against women in labour, to the extent that women have become alienated from the birth experience and the role of the midwife has been slowly but surely eroded. There are many different kinds of feminism. Some midwives are feminists, many are not, some are not sure. The sole intention of this chapter is to stimulate discussion and debate.

■ **It is assumed that you are already aware of the following:**

● The physiology of normal pregnancy and labour;

● The fundamental difference between a midwifery model and a medical model of care in labour;

- Feminist thinking in relation to gender and inequality;
- The recent changes in the provision of the maternity services.

■ Men and midwifery

The term 'male midwife' first entered the English language in the 1600s. By the 17th century, the male midwife was being called to attend a birth if surgical intervention was required. Normal labour remained within the province of the female midwife. Gradually, male midwives became more fashionable, especially among upper-class women, and men began to compete directly with female midwives for the care of women in normal labour. These male midwives were the forerunners of the modern day obstetrician (Oakley 1976).

The medical profession at this time was not interested in childbirth because of the belief that women's reproductive powers had the potential to 'pollute' and were therefore 'dangerous to society' (Oakley 1976: 32). Male midwives were regarded with disdain by 'real' doctors, but eventually, in the 1800s, midwifery was included in general medical training. At this time, women were excluded from the medical profession, and female midwives still did not have direct access to a formal training (Oakley 1976). Scientific discovery and experiment continued, and this further eroded the role of the female midwife. The medicalisation of childbirth was able to begin in earnest.

■ Women and childbirth

At the turn of the century, women's experiences of childbearing were not good. Women had frequent pregnancies, and, as a result of poverty and ill-health, many working-class women had difficult pregnancies and painful births in less than ideal conditions That being the case, it is hardly surprising that women had a real fear of childbirth and consequently wanted to give birth in hospital (Lewis 1990; Hunt & Symonds 1995).

Eventually, hospital confinement was recommended for all women (DHSS 1970). Giving birth in hospital has effectively further disempowered both women in labour and midwives, and has finally enabled doctors to take almost total control of the labour process. The increasing reliance on technology has resulted in a loss of midwifery skills and has blurred the boundaries between midwifery and obstetric practice to the extent that midwives function as obstetric nurses acting as assistants to doctors, rather than as midwives with an autonomous clinical role. Consequently, many midwives are no longer 'with women' in labour. This has resulted in the labour ward culture of the 1990s described by Hunt (Hunt & Symonds 1995), wherein women – as if on a production line – are defined and only given time by midwives depending upon the degree of dilatation of their cervix.

Many midwives appear to collude in this process (Hunt & Symonds 1995). Bartky (1990: 11–21), a feminist philosopher, suggests that such collusion arises because of what she describes as 'a divided consciousness', meaning that women, although seeing themselves as victims of an unjust system of social power, can nevertheless perceive it as being natural, inevitable and inescapable, the result being that they remain blind to the extent to which they themselves are implicated in the victimisation of other women.

Criticism of the medicalisation of childbirth by feminist writers has been considerable (Oakley 1976, 1980, 1986; Ehrenreich & English 1979; Doyal 1995; Tew 1995). They question the obstetric view that all births must be perceived as being 'at risk' until the woman has delivered and proved otherwise. This approach has resulted in the routine application of technology in labour regardless of whether women want or need it. Economics plays an important part in this. We live in a technology-driven, consumerist, capitalist society. Spallone considers that industrialised nations are 'locked into a dependent relationship with science and technology'. She is also of the view that 'the power of technology is everywhere and the interests of the privileged are tied up in it' (Spallone 1989: 91).

The modern scientific approach to childbirth came about as Western thought and medicine developed. The body was likened to a machine. This view of the body is supported by the Cartesian model, which is based on a belief in a mind/body split. Martin (1989: 54) refers to this as a 'mechanical metaphor' – the body has parts, that is, organs, which can now, in the 20th century, be replaced, as in transplant surgery. Tools – the instruments used by the surgeon (Martin 1989) – are needed to service and repair machinery. Childbirth was, by the 19th century, seen as essentially a mechanical process: medical literature referred to 'the mechanism of labour' (Donnison 1988: 59).

Obstetrics developed by replacing the female midwife's hands with male hands using a variety of tools. The female midwife was considered 'unfitted by nature for all scientific mechanical employment', and midwives therefore 'could not use obstetric instruments with advantage or precision even if they had the presumption enough to try' (Donnison 1988). The application of technology to childbirth has reached a point at which, in the 20th century, Wertz and Wertz (1989: 165) can describe childbirth in America as the 'processing of a machine, by machines and skilled technicians'. This description could equally be applied to childbirth in the UK.

During the 20th century, maternal and perinatal mortality rates have been greatly reduced, but maternal morbidity may not have been. An investigation of long-term health problems directly associated with childbirth (MacArthur *et al* 1991) reveals that, of 11 701 women surveyed, 47 per cent suffered chronic ill-health after childbirth. The problems that women reported included chronic backache, musculoskeletal problems, frequent headaches and migraine, stress incontinence, depression, anxiety and extreme tiredness. For some women, these problems were still present 9 years after giving birth. Careful reading of the study suggests that much of this modern-day ill-health can be attributed to the medicalisation of normal childbirth. Obstetricians would disagree and argue that the use of technology has made childbirth safer for both mother and baby.

Wertz and Wertz consider that obstetricians are more concerned with the baby than with the mother: 'in the eyes of medicine, the fetus is primarily a medical product, subject to medicine's quality control as it moves along the gestational assembly line' (Wertz & Wertz 1989: 242). Consequently, intervention is required to ensure the safe delivery of a healthy child regardless of the psychological or physical ill-effects it may have on the mother. In recent years, the press has been reporting cases in which High Court judges have compelled women to have caesarean sections against their will in the interests of the fetus, for example the case of Mrs S, who refused a caesarean section for religious reasons (Hewson 1996). While applying to the courts has become accepted practice in America (French 1992), it is relatively new to the UK and raises serious ethical issues, such as those of informed consent. Beverley Beech, Honorary Chair of the Association for Improvements in the Maternity Services (AIMS), in a letter to the *Times*, considers these incidents to demonstrate that obstetricians are using the courts to support an authoritarian pattern of care. She also suggests that some interventions 'are neither essential nor urgent'. She says that AIMS helps many women to deal with the 'disastrous emotional effects' caused by the over-zealous use of technology in labour (Beech 1996). Robinson (1995: 335) describes this form of suffering as 'technology iatrogenesis' – that is, the emotional damage inflicted by intervention, and this is often exacerbated by what she calls 'behavioral iatrogenesis', in which midwives and obstetricians behave badly towards women in labour. It would appear that the medicalisation of labour has resulted in the midwife, rather than being 'with woman' in labour, becoming what Donnison (1988: 209) describes as 'a machine minder to the obstetric engineer'.

Following the implementation of the Peel Report (DHSS 1970) in the 1970s, pressure groups such as the National Childbirth Trust (NCT) and AIMS set about trying to reassert women's control of the childbearing process. Tew, who started researching maternity care in the 1970s, comments that she initially had great difficulty in getting her work published because she was opposing 'the establishment' (Tew 1995: viii). Her writing presented evidence about a false use of statistics to support a system that was actually harming women and babies.

Eventually, the Winterton Report (House of Commons Health Committee 1992) was commissioned. The government wanted efficient, effective and economical maternity care. The content and nature of the report suggests that the Winterton Committee set out to serve the best interests of women as well as to address cost effectiveness. The Winterton Committee was interested in the social context of childbearing and in health inequality. It also questioned the validity of the prevailing medical model of birth. Consequently, the Winterton Report had the potential to legitimise midwifery practice, but it was a lost opportunity because much of the government's eventual response to the Report was non-committal and evasive.

The committee listened to evidence presented by many interested groups, including the Royal College of Midwives (RCM), the Royal College of Obstetricians and Gynaecologists (RCOG), the NCT and individual childbearing women who had experience of the maternity services. The Committee considered that more detailed and accurate research was required into interventions that have become commonplace in labour wards, such as induction, epidurals, electronic fetal monitoring and caesarean sections.

The report recommended that, until the results of such research were available, interventions of this nature should not be used as a matter of routine in normal labour. This was contrary to the views of the many eminent obstetricians who had given evidence to the committee.

In its written response to the Winterton Report, the RCOG argued that 'There can be no retreat from science'. The challenge, as the obstetricians appeared to see it, was to 'accommodate' technology so that 'it is used appropriately with maximum effect and detracts as little as possible from the experience of childbirth' (RCOG 1992). The Winterton Report was not implemented as it stood, but an Expert Committee was convened, chaired by Baroness Cumberlege. The resulting *Changing childbirth* report (DoH 1993) was a reformulation of Winterton, in that while it appeared to promote a greater use of midwifery skills, greater choice for women, continuity of care and wanting women to have control of the childbearing process, it still, unlike Winterton, supported the medical model of birth, which meant that midwifery would remain subject to medical knowledge and control. There has also been inadequate funding for the implementation of *Changing childbirth*, so the *status quo* remains in spite of much effort by midwives to bring about change (Rothwell 1996).

While still powerful, the medical profession does not exercise the same degree of power as in the past. In NHS trusts, doctors do not have financial control and are answerable to general managers of directorates within trusts. The Chief Executive of a trust has overall power. Remaining faithful to the medical model of birth while using a less interventionist approach to normal birth is still high on the DoH's agenda: the Clinical Standards Advisory Group's (CSAG) report (1995) suggests that standards are set for the care of women in normal labour. The NHS Executive (DoH 1996) is demanding clinical effectiveness. Trusts are struggling to demonstrate cost effectiveness and are moving towards evidence-based purchasing. The stage is set for change – to a midwifery, as opposed to an obstetric model of care. It would be kinder to women and enable the desired clinical effectiveness. However, before this can happen, midwives need to draw upon their knowledge base and rethink what constitutes normal labour.

■ Childbirth from a feminist perspective

Giving birth is stressful and painful. The clinical experience of many women in labour suggests that women can develop coping mechanisms if they are not fearful and have trust in their ability to give birth and in the person caring for them. Women also need an internal, rather than an external, locus of control if they are to be able to draw upon personal resources. Ideally, giving birth should increase a woman's self-esteem and give her a sense of satisfaction. Giving birth is an emotional experience. Success in giving birth depends upon both physiological and psychological well-being and can only be personally evaluated because it is a subjective experience. Rowe (1997), a clinical psychologist/psychoanalyst, supports this view in that she considers that, contrary to popular belief, reality does not go on outside ourselves but inside our heads, meaning that each person constructs his or her own reality. Rowe also considers that emotion is not separate from cognition but is necessary in order to give meaning to our experiences. Savage (1986: 18) acknowledges that, through talking to women, she came to realise that her advice to women in labour had sometimes not been in that woman's best interests because she had interfered with the woman's own perceptions of her labour. If seen in this light, it becomes apparent that the present culture of childbirth does not work for women but against them.

Technology has become intrusive. However, women – and indeed many midwives – appear to need the reassurance it seems to provide, despite the lack of concrete evidence of its value. Childbirth is exclusive to women, yet it is controlled by different groups of men – politicians, lawyers, trust managers, obstetricians, anaesthetists, microbiologists and paediatricians. There are a small number of women within these groups, but collectively each group expresses a masculine view of childbirth. For example, Felicity Reynolds, a professor of obstetric anaesthesia, is quoted in the *Daily Mail* newspaper as saying that 'mothers should be demanding new low dose epidural injections... which are the only effective analgesia for labour pains'. She considers that women are often unaware 'that pethidine does not work' and that midwives are under the misapprehension that it does because 'it makes women drowsy and less troublesome. They can give it themselves and it is cheap' (Hope 1997: 31). Reynolds is promoting the medical model of birth and at the same time denigrating midwifery practice. On the other hand, if a woman in one of these groups chooses to step outside the collective view in the interests of women, she will be severely dealt with. As an example, consider what happened to the female obstetric consultant Wendy Savage when she questioned the notion that pregnancy can be normal only in retrospect. The way in which she was treated by colleagues led her to explore the question 'Who controls childbirth?' (Savage 1986).

From a feminist perspective, the whole of childbirth is subject to patriarchal control. Dinnerstein (1987) considers that childbirth has the potential to empower women only if women take control of the childbearing process. Firestone (1979), however, took a completely different view. She was a revolutionary, radical feminist who considered childbearing, because of patriarchal control of both childbirth and childrearing, to be the root cause of women's oppression. Firestone thought that reproductive technologies in the hands of women would be the key to women's liberation because 'test tube' babies would remove the need for women to bear children. Unfortunately, reproductive technologies have remained firmly in the hands of men (Corea 1988). Firestone displayed a certain naivety in thinking that women would be allowed to take control of what was, then, a new science. It also did not seem to occur to Firestone that they could be used to oppress rather than liberate women. Corea constructs a convincing argument to demonstrate how the reproductive technologies, rather than liberating women, have added to women's reproductive problems (Corea 1988).

Greer considers that enormous pressures are put upon women to make them conform to the masculine view of the birthing process. Consequently, any woman 'who demands the right to make her own decisions will find herself conducting a running battle with health professionals' (Greer 1984: 10). Figes, a modern day feminist, considers obstetrics and increasing technology to mean that 'mothers are more likely to blame themselves if anything goes wrong' (Figes 1995: 84). She also highlights the difficulties women encounter in trying to steer a course between the medical model and the 'natural childbirth movement'. Oakley (1980) makes the important point that childbirth itself is not inherently oppressive, but rather that the male domination of the process has made it become so.

Feminist theory offers a fresh, alternative analysis of the problems that face both women in labour and midwives. A feminist critique of care in labour is not about natural childbirth at all costs. It does not seek to abandon the use of reason and logic. The appropriate application of technology for women with a history of medical, gynaecological or obstetric problems has undoubtedly saved the lives of women and babies, but its routine use in normal labour has alienated women from the birth experience. The term 'natural' childbirth is not a good one. Nature left to its own devices can create havoc. The preferred term is 'active' birth. It creates a mental picture of a woman actively giving birth rather than being delivered. She is alert and in control, liberated from the fear of childbirth. Scientific thinking should be able to assist in this process, but it cannot in its present mode. Rowe (1997) is of the view that what she describes as powerful forces, fear, avarice and the desire for power have affected scientific thinking, and, rather than a search for truth, science has become more a quest for the fulfilment of personal desires. She uses this argument to explain why psychotherapy, in her view, does not work. Her argument could also be used to explain why science has failed women in normal labour.

Science prides itself on its use of logic and reasoning – rational thought, the ability to be objective. But childbirth is a subjective experience and the routine application of technology to fit, healthy women in normal labour is, surely, irrational and suggests that the forces described by Rowe are at work. A collective name for these forces could be patriarchy. Women in normal labour have become victims of what Spallone calls 'patriarchal science', that is, science that seeks to meet the needs and self-interest of men, often at the expense of women (Spallone 1989: 192).

■ Patriarchy

Feminists believe that the driving force behind a worldwide oppression of women is patriarchy. Understanding the concept of patriarchy is central to understanding the reasoning behind feminist thinking and how gender inequality is maintained. The word 'patriarchy' is derived from the Greek meaning 'rule of the father'. The sociologist Max Weber used the term to describe a particular form of household in which the father is the head (Haralambos & Holborn 1995). This is known as private patriarchy. Early radical feminists (Millett 1970) took the concept a step further, describing a public form of patriarchy, the fundamental, universal state of male dominance over women through the social structures of the society in which we live, for example government, law, education and religion. Out of these structures come other patriarchal structures, such as the media, publishing houses and organisations such as the NHS, the police and the armed forces. These structures ensure that men have control over all aspects of society, including the part women do or do not play in it. The feminist movement has campaigned relentlessly to secure for women the same rights as men, but the patriarchal control of childbirth nonetheless remains because women have, over a long period of time, been made vulnerable to the idea that a doctor in control of pregnancy and birth represents safety.

Rich gives an all-embracing definition of patriarchy as:

> a familial-social, ideological, political system in which men – by force, direct pressure, or through ritual, tradition, law and language, customs, etiquette, education, and the division of labour, determine what part women shall or shall not play, and in which the female is everywhere subsumed under the male.
>
> Rich (1977: 57)

Feminists have challenged the power of patriarchy, but it remains very powerful and all-pervasive. Hubbard describes it as being:

> completely intertwined and hidden in the ordinary truths and realities that the people who live in the society accept without question. This tends to obscure the fact that these beliefs are actively generated and furthered by members of the dominant group because they are consistent with that group's interests.
>
> (in Lowe & Hubbard 1983: 1)

Hubbard, and Rich, could have been writing about everyday life on a labour ward. Obstetric practice is completely intertwined and hidden in the ordinary everyday truths and realities of a day in the life of a labour ward. Women and midwives accept, even expect, medical intervention as a matter of course. The institution of obstetrics will continue to promote its own cause; it is in its interests to do so if it is to survive. To do this, it must promote technology and undermine both midwifery practice and women's belief in their ability to give birth without obstetric intervention.

If the obstetrician cannot be present, he or she will impose a presence through labour ward policies, protocols and guidelines. Hospital labour wards have traditions, customs and rituals. There is a language of labour that is incomprehensible to the uninitiated and certain etiquettes are observed, such as summoning a senior house officer before the registrar or consultant. Most midwives have educational backgrounds very different from those of obstetricians, and there is a definite division of labour. Obstetricians need to control midwifery practice in order to ensure that women and midwives conform to the medical model of birth. A good example of this is the time limit put on the second stage of labour. This practice persists in labour wards despite evidence suggesting that if the second stage is progressing, as demonstrated by descent of the presenting part, and the condition of both mother and baby remains satisfactory, there is no need for intervention (Sleep *et al* 1989, see also Chapter 7 in this volume).

Shorter (1983) argues that childbirth was once difficult, painful and dangerous and that this situation has been alleviated by the development of modern obstetrics. This is not entirely correct. What brought about the reduction in the maternal mortality rate was the improvement of social conditions and awareness of the need for hygiene and nutrition. The largest decrease in maternal mortality – approximately 40–50 per cent – occurred during the 1930s and 40s (Tew 1995). The introduction of sulphonamide drugs, which reduced the number of deaths resulting from sepsis, and the use of ergometrine and blood transfusions, which reduced the number of deaths due to haemorrhage (Myles 1964), played a large part in the decline of maternal mortality. This was 30 years before 'modern obstetrics' got into its stride (Tew 1995). Furthermore, doctors rather than midwives were able to appear to women to be making childbirth safer because, as men, they had access to a formal education and could take part in scientific experiment, which was denied to midwives as women. The art of midwifery was not considered scientific and therefore lacked credibility. Clarke (1994) believes that this problem remains today. Midwives now have access to a formal education and training, but the two dominant discourses of childbirth – medical and natural – remain.

Cosslett reminds us of a third discourse, so embedded in the subconscious of women that it is often overlooked: the unofficial discourse or 'old wives' tales', the oral tradition of women telling each other about childbirth. She describes them as 'unstructured, ghoulish horror stories that challenge the simple, optimistic structures of our modern myths of birth' (Cosslett 1994: 4). To a great extent, these old wives' tales have been marginalised by the medical model because, as De Vries (1993: 134) observes, 'Technology brings in its wake ideas, definitions and approaches to childbirth that supplant traditional patterns'. He asserts that formal training discounts all other sources of knowledge, including traditional midwifery and what he calls 'the unique information a client possesses (about her body, previous births and so on)'. However, the power of the oral tradition should not be underestimated because it works for the medical model of birth in that it can make women fearful.

Downe (1994) highlights the fact that midwives generally allow others, for example obstetricians, lawyers, non-midwifery managers and statisticians, to define normality for them. The probable reason for this is that the midwifery profession has been severely weakened by the profound effect of the scientific revolution on pregnancy and birth since the 1960s. Enshrined in obstetric propaganda is the belief that all women in labour are 'at risk', so midwives and women have lost sight of what constitutes a normal labour, and it is a sad truth that if you treat all women as high risk, they are inclined to become so (Oakley 1993).

Women who are not midwives (and not necessarily feminists) have long argued against the medicalisation of birth. Kitzinger's prolific writings acknowledge the wholeness of the birth experience for women. Birth, she writes:

> cannot simply be a matter of techniques for getting a baby out of one's body. It involves our relationship to life as a whole, the part we play in the order of things.
>
> (Kitzinger 1978: 27)

Cosslett (1994) acknowledges the wholeness of the birth experience for women. She describes the power of narrative to demonstrate women's feelings in relation to giving birth and draws upon the work of writers such as Doris Lessing and Fay Weldon. Cosslett examines in detail readings of women's birth stories. When women write 'from the heart', they display their inner feelings about childbirth. Descriptions of maternity hospitals conjure up images of cold, impersonal places; feelings of isolation and aloneness in an alien territory come through. Such narratives reflect the truth of Kitzinger's statement in that, for women, there is more to childbirth than simply 'pushing out' a baby. Women in labour are vulnerable and are dependent on those around them; hospitals are not the best places for women in normal labour to give birth. When giving birth, women need to feel safe and also be surrounded by those they love, people who know them as a person rather than just another woman in labour. Raven describes her experience of the hospital birth of her first child as 'draining and demeaning', whereas the home birth of her second child, although just as long and painful, was 'powerful and passionate'. She writes, 'I think of it and smile' (Raven 1997: 7).

Raphael Leff, a clinical psychoanalyst, describes birth as being 'a personal issue of emotional intimacy' with the power to arouse subconscious fantasies and fears in the woman in labour and her birth attendants (Raphael Leff 1991: 258). If we are to provide woman-centred care, we must acknowledge these subconscious, mystical aspects of giving birth. This may seem an impossible task because science has effectively demystified pregnancy and birth with interventions such as *in vitro* fertilisation techniques and ultrasound. However, even though the conscious mind may now be able to observe a much magnified ovum and sperm, or a fetus, on an ultrasound screen, irrational fantasies and fears about the birthing process remain buried in the subconscious mind.

DeVries (1993) suggests that technology is able to create a uniform culture, that is, an environment in which the routine, relentless use of technology becomes accepted as the norm, and that it will eventually make midwifery obsolete. This may not be the stated intention of obstetricians, but midwifery practice shaped by their authority is fast assuming the obstetric nurse role. Women, however, appear to think differently from DeVries. Having experienced the traumas caused by technology, many are requesting – some even demanding – a more holistic approach. The result of a series of NCT surveys on what women want from midwives and other health care professionals demonstrated that women value and want the type of care offered by midwives (Hutton 1996). Some might question the validity of this survey because there is a common belief among midwives and obstetricians that women who belong to the NCT tend to be of a certain 'type', that is, they are well-educated, middle-class women (Green *et al* 1990), and the survey is therefore unlikely to reflect the views of less well-educated working-class women. However, Green *et al* (1990) looked at this 'stereotyping' of women and discovered that there is little evidence to support the view that the needs of women are different according to their education and class. Their prospective survey of women's expectations of birth revealed that women, irrespective of education, had the same desires: to avoid drugs in labour and to have control of the childbirthing process; interestingly, it was the less-educated women who had the highest expectations of giving birth, anticipating it to be a fulfilling experience (Green *et al* 1990: 125).

The public are also questioning the medical model of birth. For example, an article in a Sunday newspaper magazine questions the routine use of Syntocinon in labour. The article considers that it is misused to the detriment of mother and baby and suggests that a change is needed in the 'overall approach to labour, away from the current, technology-driven methods' (Ashton 1996: 22) taking place in maternity hospitals today.

Once a woman enters a hospital, she is in an alien environment. This will affect her behaviour patterns and encourage her to perceive herself as a patient. A patient needs a doctor, and the midwife slips into the role of nurse. To describe her observations of the interaction between obstetrician, midwife and mother, Oakley (1993) uses the analogy of the obstetrician as the father figure, the midwife the mother and the pregnant woman the child. While *Changing childbirth* has theoretically opened the door to giving women more choice in relation to the place of birth, the majority of women (and midwives) now appear firmly to believe that hospital is the safest place in which to give birth. It will take a considerable length of time to restore women's confidence in their ability to give birth outside the hospital environment.

■ The power of language

The primary source of patriarchal control is through language (Walby 1990). The language of the labour ward is the language of obstetrics, which means that it is objective rather than subjective and reflects the masculine view of birth. It is through language that we can communicate verbally what we think and what we feel. Giles and Coupland understood the power of language when they wrote:

> Our social lives are built around the symbolic functioning of language; in our language we give life, meaning and value to our relationships, allegiances, institutions and of course to ourselves; the social conditions that structure all of these again find their shape in the language we use.
>
> (Giles & Coupland 1991)

The 1996 NCT surveys mentioned above highlighted the barrier that language creates between obstetrician and woman. More than one third of women commented that they often did not understand the language used by the obstetrician. But the obstetrician needs this barrier in order to maintain the status of expert. Society gives doctors this status. When speaking with women, midwives need to examine the language they use and the way they speak it. Tone of voice can express even more than the words used and cause the often untold distress experienced by women in labour described by Robinson (1995).

Spender (1980) argues that language is patriarchally structured, that is, made by men, for men. She considers that male language, when used to define women's work, can make women invisible; indeed, obstetrics has nearly (but not quite) made midwifery invisible, for example by moving normal birth from home to hospital. The public associates hospitals with illness. Hospitals have patients who are cared for by doctors and nurses. Midwives who work in hospitals wear a uniform that makes them indistinguishable from nurses.

Spender (1980) sees language as promoting male imagery and a masculine view of the world that puts women at a disadvantage. This argument could be applied to the language of obstetrics. A good example is the changing of the name 'labour ward' to 'delivery suite'. This is a direct response to obstetric practice. The change of name has taken away the emphasis from what women do in the ward – labour – to what obstetricians do – deliver women. This change of name has enabled the promotion of a masculine view of the labour process.

The term 'elderly primigravida' has enabled the medical profession to define a right age for first-time pregnancy and enables the categorisation of older women as being at high risk of complications and therefore needing obstetric rather than midwifery care.

Churchill considers that medical terminology is frequently used to prevent women being properly informed. Consequently, she believes that the notion of consent in childbirth ' becomes a nonsense' (Churchill 1995: 32). Because of the nature of the language used by doctors, women cannot always be expected to understand fully the exact nature and implications of a treatment being recommended. Equally, those wishing to challenge the medical model of birth can use emotive language and imagery with intent to shock. Kitzinger (1988: 17), for example, describes episiotomy as 'a crude assault', 'female mutilation' and 'abuse', whereas doctors and midwives perceive it as a useful, simple method of expediting delivery. Kitzinger portrays hospitals as a hostile environment for women, whereas the original, stated intent of hospital confinement was to make childbirth safer for women.

■ Redefining normality

Obstetrics remains male dominated. Pathologising pregnancy and birth is a very effective way of removing women's autonomy and authority. The control of childbirth is about power: the power of men over women. Whereas Freud's framework for describing human psychosexual and moral development maintains that women suffer from 'penis envy' – the Electra complex (Gross 1987: 520) – Raphael Leff considers that it is, in fact, men who are envious of women's capacity to give birth, and this has resulted in 'false assumptions, taboos, protective rituals and cultural superimpositions' which complicate the normal birth process' (Raphael Leff 1991: 258).

O'Driscoll and Meagher, in their book *Active management of labour* (1980), provide an excellent example of how male obstetricians can regiment and control women's experience of labour. They set the trend for the rigorous management of labour for many years to come. Consequently, a woman in normal labour can expect to have an amniotomy, a fetal scalp electrode applied, fetal blood sampling, a Syntocinon infusion and possibly an epidural, be urged to push prematurely in the second stage of labour, and finally have an episiotomy to expedite delivery; the third stage of labour will be actively managed and the midwife, when completing the notes, will write 'normal delivery' or 'spontaneous vertex delivery'! (See Chapter 4 in this volume for a fuller discussion of the active management of labour.)

Mavis Kirkham understood the impact of rampant technology on midwifery practice when she wrote:

> Previously all pregnancies were seen as normal until judged otherwise, a judgement initially made by the midwife. The reverse is now true, as all pregnancies now fall under medical management and are 'normal only in retrospect'. By this logic the midwife as a practitioner in her own right is defined out of existence.
>
> Kirkham (1986: 37)

Odent acknowledges that the priority of obstetrics is to control childbirth and takes no account of the normal physiology of birth. He believes that it is essential to rediscover the role of *authentic* midwives, whom he considers to be 'the only people who do not disturb the physiology of birth' (Odent 1986: 136).

As defined by Odent, the authentic midwife perceives labour in a healthy woman who has had an uncomplicated pregnancy as normal until it proves itself otherwise. The pain of normal labour is perceived as having a purpose. It tells a woman that labour has begun. As the contractions increase in length, strength and frequency, this tells both woman and midwife that labour is progressing. Pain in normal labour is very different from pain in abnormal labour. The 'silent' labour produced by epidural analgesia not only renders the pelvic floor inert and therefore interferes with the physiology of normal labour, but it can also mask the onset of abnormality. Illich (1976: 144) observed that 'as culture is medicalized, the social determinants of pain are distorted... medical civilization focuses primarily on pain as a systemic reaction that can be verified, measured, and regulated'. With the increasing medicalisation of birth involving the use of Syntocinon, the pain of labour has been distorted, and women will need some form of pain relief rather than relying on their own natural coping mechanisms.

A study of 10 702 women (Rajan 1993) shows that doctors' and midwives' observations of whether or not analgesia in labour was effective was at odds with the women's own experience. What the professionals considered to be effective pain relief, the woman considered to be poor. Illich was aware of this potential danger in relation to the experience of pain. He believes that allowing doctors to take over any traditional culture will result in doctors denying the individual experience of pain, and this will have a knock-on effect on the individual and society's attitude towards pain as a whole:

> The medical profession judges which pains are authentic... which pains have a physical base... which a psychic base, which are imagined and which are simulated. Society recognises and endorses this professional judgement. Compassion becomes an obsolete virtue. The person in pain is left with less and less social context to give meaning to the experience... .
>
> Illich (1976: 144–5)

Allowing obstetric control of the birthing process has placed childbirth in a medical rather than a social context. Consequently, the normal pain of childbirth no longer has any meaning or value. It is something to be controlled, preferably by an outside agency. Childbirth today is physically safer for both mothers and babies (Savage 1986). Therefore women are now in a position to be encouraged to take responsibility for their own labour experience. Evidence collected by Lagercrantz and Slotkin (1986) supports the view that normal labour is not harmful to most infants. They consider that the 'stress' of birth is normal and that the physiological surge of catecholamines that occurs in babies during labour is important to the neonate's survival at birth.

A woman who has had an uncomplicated pregnancy should be allowed the privacy to labour undisturbed. A confident woman who feels in control, is given freedom of position and movement and is allowed to eat and drink at will in early labour, will have a shorter, less painful labour and an easier birth (Odent 1986). Unfortunately, the medical model of birth discourages women from making this discovery (Odent 1984). This discouragement is all part of the process of attempting to control the childbirth process. Davies, like Raphael Leff (1991), is of the view that this desire to control the process of birth stems from 'a fear of birth' (Davies 1996: 285).

Mason (1996: 658) considers that midwifery has the potential to serve the best interests of mothers and babies but not while it remains subjected to medical knowledge and control. He suggests that midwives, rather than depending upon medical science, develop a public health perspective and harness biological processes to psychological and social circumstances. The research of Oakley *et al* (1996) supports this view. It confirms that there is a close link between social well-being and physical health, and highlights the importance of social support by midwives in pregnancy because it has a long-term, positive effect on the health of women and children.

In the labour ward, however, I suggest that midwifery practice continues to be controlled by and respond to obstetric practice. The extended role of the midwife has effectively blurred the boundaries between midwifery and obstetric practice, and midwives are now taking the same interventionist approach as obstetricians, thus enabling the medical control of childbirth to continue. In order to meet the needs of women and the midwifery profession, there is an urgent need for midwives, along with women, to redefine what constitutes normal labour and birth.

■ Discussion points

1. If a woman is healthy and has had an uncomplicated pregnancy, can labour be regarded as normal until it proves itself otherwise, or can labour only be seen as normal in retrospect?

2. What are the implications for mother and baby if a non-interventionist approach is used for normal labour?

3. What are the implications for risk management if labour is perceived as normal until it proves itself otherwise?

4. What are the implications for the midwifery profession if:
    a) labour is considered normal until it proves itself otherwise;
    b) labour can only be considered normal in retrospect?

■ Practice check

- What is your definition of normal labour?

- How do you establish whether labour is normal?

- How do you enable women to make informed choices?

- If a woman wishes to make a choice about the management of her labour that would not be your choice, how easy do you find it to support her?

- To what extent do you feel able to act as 'advocate' for the women in your care?

■ References

Ashton J 1996 Hard labour night and day. Mail On Sunday Review, November 17: 19–22

Bartky SL 1990 Femininity and domination: studies in the phenomenology of oppression. Routledge, London, p11–21

Beech B 1996 Letters to the Editor, Times, December 23, p15

Churchill H 1995 Perceptions of childbirth: are women properly informed? Nursing Times 91(45): 32–3

Clarke R 1994 But is it art? Nursing Standard 8(42): 50

Clinical Standards Advisory Group 1995 Women in normal labour. HMSO, London

Corea G 1988 The mother machine. Women's Press, London

Cosslett T 1994 Women writing childbirth: modern discourses of motherhood. Manchester University Press, Manchester, p4

Davies S 1996 Divided loyalties: the problem of normality. British Journal of Midwifery 4(6): 285–6

Department of Health 1993 Changing childbirth. Report of the Expert Maternity Group, 1 and 11. HMSO, London

Department of Health 1996 Promoting clinical effectiveness: a framework for action in and through the NHS. NHS Executive

Department of Health and Social Security, Standing Maternity and Midwifery Advisory Committee 1970 Domiciliary midwifery and maternity bed needs (Chairman J Peel). HMSO, London

DeVries RG 1993 A cross-national view of the status of midwives. In Riska E, Wegar K (eds) Gender, work and medicine. Sage, London, p134

Dinnerstein D 1987 The rocking of the cradle and the ruling of the world. Women's Press, London

Donnison J 1988 Midwives and medical men. Historical Publications, London, p59, 209

Downe S 1994 How average is normality? British Journal of Midwifery 2(7): 303–4

Doyal L 1995 What makes women sick? Macmillan, London

Ehrenreich B, English D 1979 For her own good. Pluto Press, London

Figes K 1995 Because of her sex. Pan Books, London, p84

Firestone S 1979 The dialectic of sex: the case for feminist revolution. Women's Press, London

French M 1992 The war against women. Penguin, Harmondsworth

Giles H, Coupland H 1991. Cited in Hewison A 1993 The language of labour: an examination of the discourses of childbirth. Midwifery 9, p225

Green JM, Kitzinger JV, Coupland VA 1990 Stereotypes of childbearing women: a look at some evidence. Midwifery 6: 125–32

Greer G 1984 Sex and destiny. The politics of human fertility. Secker & Warburg, London, p10

Gross RD 1987 Psychology: the science of mind and behaviour. Edward Arnold, London, p520

Haralambos M, Holborn M 1995 Sociology: themes and perspectives, 4th edn. Collins Educational, London

Hewson B 1996 Court-ordered caesareans: an unnecessary development. British Journal of Midwifery 4(10): 509–10

Hope J 1997 Conned in childbirth. Daily Mail, January 3: 31

House of Commons Health Committee 1992 Sessions 1991–1992 Second report, maternity services (Chairman N Winterton). HMSO, London

Hunt S, Symonds A 1995 The social meaning of midwifery. Macmillan, Basingstoke

Hutton E 1996 What women want from midwives, obstetricians, general practitioners, health visitors and anaesthetists. National Childbirth Trust, Glasgow

Illich I 1976 Limits to medicine. Penguin, London, Ch 3, pp144–5

Kirkham M. (1986) In Webb C (ed.) Feminist practice in women's health care. John Wiley, Chichester, p37

Kitzinger S 1978 The experience of childbirth, 4th edn. Penguin, London, p27

Kitzinger S (ed.) 1988 The midwife challenge. Pandora, London, p17

Lagercrantz H, Slotkin TA 1986 The 'stress' of being born. Scientific American 254(4): 100–7

Lewis J 1990 Mothers and maternity policies in the twentieth century. In Garcia J, Kilpatrick R, Richards M (eds) The politics of maternity care. Clarendon Press, Oxford, Ch 1

Lowe M, Hubbard R (eds) 1983 Woman's nature. Pergamon Press, New York, p1

MacArthur C, Lewis M, Knox EG 1991 Health after childbirth. HMSO, London

Martin E 1989 The woman in the body, 2nd edn. Open University Press, Milton Keynes, p57

Mason J 1996 Science for midwives. British Journal of Midwifery 4(12): 657–9

Millett K 1970 Sexual politics. Virago, London

Myles MF 1964 A textbook for midwives, 5th edn. E & S Livingstone, Edinburgh

Oakley A 1976 Wisewoman and medicine man. In Mitchell J, Oakley A (eds) The rights and wrongs of women, Ch 1. Pelican Books, London

Oakley A 1980 Women confined. Martin Robertson, Oxford

Oakley A 1986 The captured womb. Basil Blackwell, Oxford

Oakley A 1993 Birth as a 'normal' process. Essays on women, medicine and health. Edinburgh University Press, Edinburgh, pp124–38

Oakley A, Hickey D, Rajan L 1996 Social support in pregnancy: does it have long-term effects? Journal of Reproductive and Infant Psychology 14: 7–22

Odent M 1984 Birth reborn: what childbirth should be. Souvenir Press, London

Odent M 1986 Primal health. Century Paperbacks, London, pp132, 136

O'Driscoll K, Meagher D 1980 Active management of labour. WB Saunders, Philadelphia

Rajan L 1993 Perceptions of pain and pain relief in labour: the gulf between experience and observation. Midwifery 9: 136–45

Raphael Leff J 1991 Psychological processes of childbearing. Chapman & Hall, London, p258

Raven S 1977 No place like home. Sunday Telegraph, February 23: 7

Rich A 1977 Of woman born: motherhood as experience and institution. Virago, London, pp57, 129

Robinson J 1995 Behavioural iatrogenesis. British Journal of Midwifery 3(6): 335

Rothwell H 1996 Changing childbirth. Changing nothing. Midwives   109(1306): 291–4

Rowe D 1997 The comforts of unreason. In Kennard D, Small N (eds) Living together. Quartet Books, London

Royal College of Obstetricians and Gynaecologists 1992 Response to the Report of the House of Commons Health Committee on Maternity Services. RCOG, London

Savage W 1986 A Savage enquiry, who controls childbirth? Virago, London, p18

Shorter E 1983 A history of women's bodies. Allen Lane, London

Sleep J, Roberts J, Chalmers I 1989 Care during the second stage of labour. In Chalmers I, Enkin M, Keirse MJNC (eds) Effective care in pregnancy and child-birth, vol. 2, Childbirth. Oxford University Press, Oxford

Spallone P 1989 Beyond conception: the new politics of reproduction. Macmillan Education, Basingstoke, pp191–2

Spender D 1980 Man made language. Routledge, London

Tew M 1995 Safer childbirth? A critical history of maternity care, 2nd edn. Chapman & Hall, London

Walby S 1990 Theorizing patriarchy. Basil Blackwell, Oxford

Wertz RW, Wertz DC 1989 Lying-in: a history of childbirth in America, 2nd edn. Yale University Press, New York

■ Suggested further reading:

Appignanesi R, Zarate O 1992 Freud for beginners. Icon Books, Cambridge

Raphael-Leff J 1993 Pregnancy. The inside story. Sheldon Press, London

Sydie RA 1987 Natural women, cultured men: a feminist perspective on sociological theory. Open University Press, Milton Keynes

Tong R 1989 Feminist thought. Routledge, London

Ussher J 1989 The psychology of the female body. Routledge, London

Index

145